CATATONIA

CATATONIA

K.L. KAHLBAUM

With an Introduction by
George Mora, M.D.

The Johns Hopkins University Press
Baltimore, Maryland

Prepared under the Special Foreign Currency Program of
The National Library of Medicine,
National Institutes of Health, Public Health Service,
U.S. Department of Health, Education and Welfare,
and published for
THE NATIONAL LIBRARY OF MEDICINE
pursuant to an agreement with
THE NATIONAL SCIENCE FOUNDATION, WASHINGTON, D.C.,
by
THE ISRAEL PROGRAM FOR SCIENTIFIC TRANSLATIONS,
JERUSALEM, ISRAEL

Copyright © 1973 by The Johns Hopkins University Press
All rights reserved

Translated from the German *Die Katatonie oder das Spannungsirresein*
by
Y. Levij, M.D. and T. Pridan, M.D.

The Johns Hopkins University Press, Baltimore, Maryland 21218

Library of Congress Catalog Card Number 72-9960
ISBN 0-8018-1483-9

Composed and printed in Israel by Keter Press, Jerusalem

Contents

Introduction to the English Translation *by G. Mora* vii
Introduction   1
Chapter One.   Preliminary Definitions of Criteria and Medical
                 Case Histories   7
Chapter Two.   Symptomatology 29
Chapter Three. Etiology. 53
Chapter Four. Pathological Anatomy 59
Chapter Five. Diagnosis 83
Chapter Six.   Prognosis. 87
Chapter Seven. Therapy. 93
Subject Index 97
Author Index 101

INTRODUCTION TO THE ENGLISH TRANSLATION
by George Mora, M.D.

I. Kahlbaum's Life and Work

Karl Ludwig Kahlbaum was born on December 28, 1828 in Dresden. He studied medicine at the universities of Königsberg, Würtzburg and Leipzig, and received a medical degree in Berlin with a thesis on the intestinal tract of birds, *"De avium tractus alimentari anatomia et histologia nonnulla,"* in 1854. Two years later he became an assistant to Dr. Bernhardi in the mental hospital of Allenberg in Wehlau, East Prussia, where he showed the greatest interest in the treatment of mental patients.

After several years of study, he became "Privatdozent" at the University of Königsberg with the monograph, "The Classification of Mental Illnesses and the Division of Emotional Disturbances" (Danzig, 1863). Three years later Kahlbaum published an important study on sensorial delusions. While in Königsberg he succeeded in establishing courses in psychiatry for medical students.

Because of some difficulties, Kahlbaum decided to leave the university in 1866 and to accept a position of assistant at the Reimer Sanitarium for the treatment of mental disturbances in Görlitz. His outstanding organizational qualities shortly afterward led to his appointment as director of that institution, where he remained until his death.

Among the innovations which Kahlbaum introduced at the Reimer Sanitarium were a special ward which soon became well-known, a "Pädagogium" (or educational facility for abnormal youngsters), and an excellent program of occupational therapy for patients in the stage of remission. Moreover, he trained a number of non-professionals, such as teachers, to be of assistance to young patients. Kahlbaum never lost sight of the concept of the whole person in treating anyone, and his case histories are outstanding.

In the meantime, the wealth of the clinical material available to him provided impetus for continuing research. Kalhbaum planned to devote a series of monographs to the most important clinical syndromes, which he had described in his 1863 volume on the classification of mental illnesses. Only two such monographs, however, were published: one on hebephrenia by his pupil Hecker in 1871[1], and one on catatonia which Kahlbaum wrote and published in 1874. Among his later writings are a monograph on "The Clinical-Diagnostic Viewpoint in Psychopathology" (1878), studies on cyclic insanity (1882), on neurological and emotional disorders in youngsters (1885) and on clinical forms of moral insanity (1885). In 1890 he addressed the International Congress of Medicine in Berlin on the theme of "dipsomania."

While these publications brought Kahlbaum considerable recognition in professional circles, it is less well known today that he also wrote many manuscripts in the fields of botany, zoology, mineralogy, paleontology, astronomy, and anthropology, which were not published. As one of the earliest supporters of scientific anthropology, Kahlbaum was especially influenced by Goethe, Kant, the naturalist Linné, and the pathologist Virchow. He was also interested in music and cultivated art.

Of liberal political ideas, Kahlbaum was friendly with German liberals and did not hesitate to disagree with Bismarck. In religion he maintained his devoted piety to his end. Always interested in traveling, he particularly liked the trip to Helgoland, at times in company with his patients. This is easily understandable in considering that he often ate and spent much time with his patients and his staff. Ewald Hecker (1843–1909), Kahlbaum's associate at the Reimer Sanitarium, became a close friend and a communion of ideas developed between them.

A number of Kahlbaum's pupils acquired prominence. Unfortunately, he was never offered a professorship in a medical school, although he made efforts to keep up with scientific developments: i.e., in 1875 he took a year off to study pathological anatomy and histology in Prague and Vienna. Kahlbaum died on April 15, 1899.

II. The State of Psychiatry in the Mid-Nineteenth Century

In order to understand the significance of Kahlbaum's work, it is necessary to present a concise picture of the development of psychiatry in the second part of the 19th century, especially in regard to methodology and philosophy of mental illness.

The field of psychiatry, *per se*, is generally considered to begin at the end of the 18th century, as the result of two interrelated trends: first, the humanitarian urge to provide independent facilities for the mentally ill (instead of abandoning them or putting them in institutions together with other outcasts of society, such as the physically handicapped, paupers and criminals, of whom people were ashamed); and, second, emergence of an interest and scientific approach in studying the course of mental illnesses. Underlying this basic change in orientation was a novel notion of man liberated from theological preoccupations and confident in his newly discovered potential to create a better and more rational society. Based on sensism (i.e., on a view of man built from the senses "below" rather than from the reason "above"), this trend had resulted in the philosophy of French ideology and of the *"Encyclopédie"* which appealed to the liberal ideas of progressive minds throughout Europe.

To be sure, mental illness had been recognized long before the advent of the Enlightenment. Attitudes toward mental disorders can be found in every society, even at the pre-literate level, and are explainable on the basis of autochthonous concepts of the mind and of reality by and large. In the context of the Western civilization, at least from Hippocrates on, notions about mental illness are inseparable from systems of classification of diseases. This is certainly true up to the 17th century, when mental disturbances were considered to be intrinsic disorders of the body–mind unity traditionally held, through the Aristotelian and Christian traditions.

Déscartes, as is known, had split that unity and from then on, throughout the 17th and the 18th century, a number of abnormal mental symptoms and conditions had been described. In contrast to a prevailing concept of a "homme-machine" in medicine—be this founded on mechanical, physical, or chemical bases—such mental aberrations tended to be viewed as caused by factors casually and empirically observed, lacking a normative notion of average mental functioning in its developmental sequence. In the attempt to put some order in this field, mental diseases came to be classified on the basis of their external manifestations, taking as a model the system of classification introduced in botany by the Swedish naturalist, Carl von Linné. Needless to say, the various classifications of mental disorders of that period —from that Felix Platter in 1602, to that of Paolo Zacchia in 1621, of Robert Burton also in 1621, of Thomas Willis in 1667, up to that of Thomas Sydenham in 1685, of Boissier de Sauvage in 1731, and of William Cullen in 1769—represent a hybrid conglomerate of brilliant anticipations of later clinical discoveries and of centuries-old superstitious ideas[2].

Yet, the epistemology of science indicates that such a classifactory stage is a necessary step toward a more critical approach to scientific inquiry. Collective, and even individual, psychological unconscious motives are not alien to any classificatory system, as shown some years ago by Henri Ellenberger in a brilliant paper on the illusions of psychiatric classifications[3].

The fact is that in the years between the end of the 18th century and the beginning of the 19th century, a new humanitarian approach to the care and treatment of the mentally ill was introduced almost at the same time, yet independently, in Florence by Vincenzo Chiarugi, in Paris by Philippe Pinel, in York, England, by William Tuke, and in the United States by Benjamin Rush. With the exception of Tuke, a layman, the other three (physicians) each left a treatise on psychiatry. Chiarugi combined a rationalistic orientation with anatomopathological reports and pioneering humanitarian insights. Pinel is noted for his thorough clinical descriptions and progressive liberal views of man. In Rush the influence of the English empirical school is overshadowed by the melioristic view of man in the newly established American democracy.

Of the three, Pinel's treatise represented the beginning of the flourishing French school of psychiatry, the success of which was probably related to the preeminence of French culture over the rest of Europe in the realm of the humanities, philosophy and science, supported by a centuries-old central government and by a network of solid institutions. In the wave of Pinel's reform, his favored pupil, Jean Etienne Esquirol, who clearly described hallucinations and "monomania" (i.e., insanity related to a particular idea), wrote the first systematic textbook of psychiatry and was instrumental in the passing of proper legislation for the mentally ill. Others greatly contributed to clinical progress: G. Ferrus, F. Voisin, and E. Seguin in regard to mental deficiency; E. J. Georget to legal psychiatry; J.P. Falrét and J. Baillarger to "circular insanity" (i.e., manic-depressive psychosis) and J. Moreau de Tours to the subjective symptomatology related to drugs. Unquestionably, however, the main accomplishment of the French school was the recognition of dementia paralytica as a separate disease by L. F. Calmeil and A. L. Bayle in the 1820's, which had a tremendous impact on the whole field of psychiatry. The British school remained essentially empirical, that is, dedicated to practical matters, mainly through R. Hill's and J. Conolly's movement of "no restraint" and J. C. Prichard's notion of "moral insanity", which had much relevance for legal psychiatry. Common to both British and American early 19th century psychiatry was the philosophy of "moral treatment", namely, of a warm atmosphere in a small mental hospital under the guidance of a dedicated superintendent.

In Germany the psychiatry of the time was heavily influenced by speculative notions and the split between the two contrasting schools of the "Psychikern" and of the "Somatiker": the first (J. Heinroth, J. C. Reil, K. Ideler, F. E. Beneke, E. Feuchtersleben) attributing mental disorders to psychological causes, and the second (F. Nasse, M. Jacobi, W. Griesinger) to organic causes. Regardless of differences in ideology, the attitude toward the mentally ill was still largely authoritarian, when not coercive, only highlighted by pioneering flashes of insight, such as the beneficial effect of sudden shocks and of theatrical performances.

Around the middle of the century, medicine came to take an increasingly physicochemical orientation, in the assumption that biological processes would be ultimately explained on that basis. Impetus toward this trend derived from the discovery of a definite etiology for a number of diseases, which led to the belief that mental diseases, similarly, were due to specific causes. From this perspective, the isolation of the three-stage clinical course of general paralysis—a typical expression of clear French rationalism—soon became the model to be followed in the identification of other mental illnesses. This trend was facilitated by the renown of the above-mentioned French clinical school and, also, by the universality of French language and culture.

By the time Kahlbaum became interested in psychiatry, in the late 1850's, the attention of many clinicians was progressively attracted by the manifestations of a condition characterized by diminution of activity, up to apathy, disorders in the formulation of thoughts, even to the point of fixation of absurd ideas, acute or insidious onset often at an early age and responding to hospital treatment only on a limited basis. The English, J. Haslam, G. Burrows, the German W. Griesinger, the French J. Baillarger, the Belgian Guislain and others, had brought scattered evidence of this clinical picture[4]. Finally, in his 1852 textbook, *Traité Théorique et Pratique des Maladies Mentales*[5], B. Morel called this condition "*démence precoce*" (dementia praecox) because of its early beginning and its unfavorable prognosis (as traditionally conveyed by the word "dementia"). Moreover, it appeared to many that such a condition followed a well-defined pattern characterized by stages and symptoms.

III. Kahlbaum's Clinical Contribution to Psychiatry

Actually, before his monograph on catatonia in 1874, Kahlbaum had already hinted at the clinical picture just described in his volume on the classification of mental illnesses of 1863. The importance of his approach in the comprehension of mental diseases consisted in describing them as temporary symptomatological patterns rather than as specific types of diseases. To clarify the matter further, Kahlbaum's pupil Hecker wrote in 1871[1] that to consider these symptomatological patterns as diseases would be the same as to consider, in somatic medicine, headache, chest pain, and abdominal pain as disease entities.

All this represented a fundamental change in the traditional understanding of mental disorders on several grounds. First, these symptomatological patterns came to be viewed as developmental stages of a "unitary psychosis". The concept of "unitary psychosis" had been brought forward by Griesinger under the influence of his teacher, E. Zeller, and had acquired momentum in the writings of H. Neumann around the 1850's[6], showing that insanity passes through the stages of melancholia, mania, amentia, and ends in dementia. Second, from this perspective, it was not necessary to wait for the discovery of the anatomopathological substratum of each disease, as the emphasis was to be placed on symptomatological patterns, rather than on diseases. Third, and as a logical consequence of the above, the main task of psychiatry had to consist of building its "empirical" foundations as a clinical" discipline on the basis of the findings presented by the patients.

With this in mind, Kahlbaum divided his book on the classification of mental disorders into three parts. In the first part he reviewed the psychiatric classifications previously published, in the second he presented in detail his own classification. In the third part Kahlbaum attempted a comparison between his classification and the previous ones and elaborated on some general considerations.

For the purpose of this introduction, it is enough to mention that Kahlbaum's classification consisted of five groups: 1) *"vesanias"* i.e., idiopathic of mental life affecting the more of less complete extent of psychic life, divided into "vesania typica" (essentically a progressively deteriorating condition as described by Neumann) and in to "vesania progressiva" (mainly the general paresis described by Bayle and Calmeil); 2) *"vecordias"*, i.e., idiopathic disturbances of mental life with limitation of the extent of the symptoms, beginning after puterty, divided into "dysthymia" (a term coined by Kahlbaum to indicate the emotional disorder traditionally called melancholia), "paranoia" (an intellectual disorder leading to to distorted ideation) and "diastrephia" (a disorder in the realm of will and performance); 3) *"dysphrenias"*, i.e., sympathic and symptomatic mental disturbances, developing in connection with a specific physiologic or pathologic bodily condition, characterized by a total illness of psychic life and mixture of the symptoms, and divided into the three forms of "nervosa", "chymosa", (i.e., affecting the vegetative system) and "sexualis"; 4) *"neophrenias"*, i.e., disturbances acquired before, with, or shortly after birth, characterized by a lack of psychological content in the manifestations of life; 5) *"paraphrenias"*, i.e., disturbances appearing in connection with one of the periods of transition of biological development (such as adolescence).

Historically, Kahlbaum's classification is the first attempt systematically to order mental disorders on the basis of the preeminence of symptomatological patterns. It is a pity that, for a variety of reasons—primarily Kahlbaum's lack of academic status in a leading university—the novelty and value of this new classification had to wait many years to be recognized.

As mentioned above, the clinical picture described as *"démence precoce"* by Morel bears many similarities with the description of *"vesania atonita"*, a category of *"vesania typica"* in his 1863 monograph on classification. Later on, in 1866, Kahlbaum described this condition in his lectures at the University of Königsberg. Finally, in 1869, he called it "catatonia" (from the Greek "to stretch tightly") for the first time in a scientific meeting in Innsbruck. Thus, his monograph on "Catatonia or Tension Insanity", represented the culmination of an idea which was in gestation for at least ten years.

In brief, the 104 page monograph on catatonia is divided into seven chapters, in which twenty-six case histories are presented. The first chapter is devoted to preliminary general considerations of the clinical course of the cases; the second to symptomatology and clarification of the specific psychic and somatic symptom-complexes (a term indicating a constellation of symptoms appearing together and related to each other); the third and the fourth to an analysis and critical observation of the etiological determinants and of the anatomical and histological findings of this disease; the fifth and the sixth to a presentation of basic data concerning its diagnosis and prognosis; the seventh, finally, to considerations related to its therapy. In general, the text is clear and effective, though at times terms derived from the Greek need to be explained.

For Kahlbaum, catatonia ("vesania catatonica") was a malignant "symptom-complex" characterized by psychotic negativism, catalepsy, mutism, steoreotypes and verbigeration (a word coined by him) and somatic disturbances (muscular symptoms). No longer satisfied, as previous nosologists, with identifying psychic symptoms in their symptomatological context, he aimed at understanding how the existing "symptom-complexes" emerge and interrelate to each other. Thus, in retrospect, his greatest contribution in, first, developing a systematic form of a disease process for a group of symptoms thus far considered heterogeneous; and, second, in having described the various stages of this disease as meaningful sequences of the same process.

The two concepts are, obviously, interrelated, inasmuch as clinical pictures hitherto considered isolated and, thus independent, are considered, instead, as successive steps of the same entity. Specifically, Kahlbaum described an initial episode of short duration of muscular abnormalities, i.e., "tension-spasm insanity" (not unlike the somatic component of the paralytical phenomena of the general paresis of the insane), characterized by the immobile posture of the flexibilitas cerea and eventually turning into hyperkinetic phenomena. This first insidious stage, corresponding to the traditional "melancholia atonita", is followed by a "stage of exaltation", punctuated by loquaciousness and pathos up to the level of extasis. Finally, through recurrent intervals of passivity and exaltation, the "stage of confusion" is reached, which ends in the complete dementia of the "defect stage".

In essence, Kahlbaum's monograph, by systematically isolating and carefully describing a clinical pattern of related symptoms in a developmental sequence, represented the best contribution of the concept of "unitary psychosis". Such a concept, clearly stated by H. Neumann (1859), was also at the base of the notion of the "*folie circulaire*" described in 1854 by J. P. Falrét as an intermittent disorder of a unitary process of various outcome, as well as of the "*folie à forme double*" (1854) of J. G. Baillarger. Interestingly enough, in his study Kahlbaum coined the word "cyclothymia" (which has since remained in the psychiatric nomenclature) to describe such a clinical notion, in which the emphasis lies in the symptomatological pattern rather than in the concept of a disease entity.

Moreover, the concept of "unitary psychosis" was also basic to the organicistic school—best represented by W. Griesinger's *Mental Pathology and Therapeutics* (1845)[7]—according to which the various mental symptoms were expressions of a pathological process in the nervous system which necessarily followed a definite course. Kahlbaum, like his contemporaries, was convinced that ultimately the etiology of catatonia lay in an anatomicopathological change in the brain; hence his belief that patients could die of catatonia, which has not been substantiated by the facts.

IV. Kahlbaum's Importance in the History of Psychiatry

At this point, it is time to attempt to assess Kahlbaum's position—especially in regard to catatonia—in the history of psychiatry.

Ten years ago, in a short but clear monograph on Kahlbaum published under the direction of the distinguished medical historian Professor E. Ackerknecht, R. Katzenstein stated that "Kahlbaum was the first German psychiatrist who systematically tried to elaborate the forms of mental diseases from the pure clinical viewpoint"[8]. Kahlbaum himself was aware of having broken new ground when he stated in the introduction to his monograph: "Such a first discovery [of catatonia] was the recognition of an entirely novel kind of psychiatric form of disease according to a hitherto unused method of definition, which we may call the clinical method, as opposed to the former methods working according to uniform psychological or unilaterally somatic principles"[9].

Unquestionably, Kahlbaum's lasting merit has been the focusing on the course of the disease, rather than on the cross-section approach used by the French authors in describing the above-mentioned clinical entities. As Katzenstein puts it, "the idea that the knowledge of the course of the disease may bring deeper insights into the different value of apparently similar clinical pictures has become the basis for all successive research"[10]. And W. De Boor, in a book on psychiatric nosology in Germany from Kahlbaum on, stated that "this knowledge has become the foundation for all further research and determines even today to a large extent the diagnostic methods of clinical psychiatry"[11].

According to Zilboorg, "after Kahlbaum's and Hecker's descriptions, a period of quiescence of erratic ideas seems to have set in German psychiatry; it lasted for about twenty years and culminated in the appearance of the monumental work of Kraepelin"[12]. As a matter of fact, during that time the French Séglas and Chaslin repeated the argument presented earlier by J. P. Falrét that Kahlbaum's attempt to differentiate catatonia on the basis of clinical observations had not been successful, inasmuch as in his monograph he had given the history of a symptom or a group of symptoms rather than a genuine and distinct form of mental disease [13]. Similar argument was brought forward by the Viennese Meynert, while, among the Germans, Schule was among the first to recognize the importance of Kahlbaum's work[14].

It is unfortunate that, in addition to Kahlbaum's lack of academic status, his difficult style further contributed to the resistance in accepting his new terminology. His pupil Hecker had alluded to the same problem in the obituary of Kahlbaum in

1899[15]. For Adolf Meyer, Kahlbaum's writings "required the digestion of too many new terms, new ideas, and new facts"[16]. C. Neisser, who highly praised Kahlbaum in a critical study[17], indicated that the novelty of his clinical approach may have been overshadowed by the difficulty posed by the new terminology. In contrast to this stands the vividness of the presentation of the case histories, which greatly impressed S. E. Jelliffe, the early American psychoanalyst and psychiatric historian[18].

In line with Zilboorg's comment, essentially Kahlbaum's importance in the history of psychiatry, that is, his definition of the concept of catatonia, is directly related to the success of Kraepelin's ideas. It is well known that Kraepelin's classification of mental diseases in his textbook, which first appeared in 1883 when he was 27, was based on the heterogeneous approach to classification typical of that period. By the time his textbook reached the fifth edition in 1896, Kraepelin had introduced his own classification of mental diseases of thirteen categories essentially based on etiology and symptomatology. In addition, he added as a sub-group, utilizing the two hitherto neglected dimensions of age of onset and course, Hecker's "hebephrenia", Kahlbaum's "catatonia", and paranoia. In the same edition the term "dementia praecox" occurred for the first time as applied to a "group" of diseases[19].

From then on, regardless of the progress in the classification of the later editions of Kraepelin's textbook, catatonia remained intrinsic to the concept of dementia praecox and, later, of schizophrenia, considered by him as leading to progressive deterioration, in contrast to the more benign manic-depressive psychosis. Kraepelin was certainly well aware of Kahlbaum's importance in psychiatry. In his monograph, *One Hundred Years of Psychiatry,* published in 1921, he stated that Kahlbaum "was the first to stress the necessity of juxtaposing the condition of the patient, his transitory symptoms, and the basic pattern underlying his disease". And later on, "it seems that the right pattern has been discovered and that patient work will bring us ever nearer to our goal".[20]

Indeed, research on catatonia has continued uninterrupted from the days of Kahlbaum. In 1930 there appeared in Paris a monograph by H. de Jong and H. Baruk on experimental catatonia[21], i.e., a catatonic condition achieved in animals through use of bulbocapnine, an alkaloid derived from "corydalis cava". In retrospect, this may be viewed as the beginning of the research on experimental psychoses which has gained momentum in recent years.

Clinically, catatonia has continued to be investigated from the psychodynamic as well as from the phenomenological perspective. Moreover, the 19th century notion of "unitary psychosis" (to which, as seen above, catatonia in its various stages greatly contributed) has become relevant again to today's attempts toward unifying human behavior[22,23,24]. Therefore, it appears very timely to present an English translation of Kahlbaum's main work to a larger audience on the eve of the centenary of its appearance.

The present translation is one of a series of classics in the history of medicine funded through the International Programs Division of the National Library of Medicine in collaboration with the Ad Hoc Committee on Historical Translations of the American Association for the History of Medicine.

The author also wishes to express his appreciation to Dr. Ihsan A. Karaagac of San Francisco, California, who originally prepared some notes on Kahlbaum's life and work, and helped to call attention to the importance of his book on catatonia.

Poughkeepsie, New York
March, 1973

George Mora, M.D.

REFERENCES TO THE INTRODUCTION TO THE ENGLISH TRANSLATION

1. HECKER, E. Die Hebephrenie. *Archiv für pathologische Anatomie und Physiologie und für klinische Medizin,* 1871, **25**, 202.
2. MENNINGER, K. (with MAYMAN, M. and PRUYSER, P.) *The Vital Balance.* New York, Viking, 1963. Appendix, pp. 419–489.
3. ELLENBERGER, H. Les illusions de la classification psychiatrique. *Evolution Psychiatrique,* 1963, **28**, 221–242.
4. ARNDT, E. Ueber die Geschichte der Katatonie. *Centralblatt für Nervenheilkunde und Psychiatrie,* 1902, **XXV**, 81–121.
5. MOREL, B. A. *Traité théorique et pratique des maladies mentales.* Paris, Baillère, 1852.
6. NEUMANN, H. *Lehrbuch der Psychiatrie.* Erlangen, Enke, 1859.
7. GRIESINGER, W. *Mental Pathology and Therapeutics.* Eng. Tr., London, Sydenham Society, 1867. (Repr. New York, Hafner, 1965). (Original German edition, 1845).
8. KATZENSTEIN, R. Karl Ludwig Kahlbaum und sein Beitrag zur Entwicklung der Psychiatrie. *Zürcher medizingeschichtliche Abhandlungen,* New Series, No. 14, Zurich, Juris, 1963.
9. KAHLBAUM, K. L. *Catatonia.* Eng. Tr. Introd. p. vii.
10. KATZENSTEIN, R., *op. cit.* p. 35.
11. DE BOOR, W. *Psychiatrische Systematik—ihre Entwicklung in Deutschland seit Kahlbaum.* Berlin, Springer, 1954, p. 6.
12. ZILBOORG, G. *A History of Medical Psychology.* New York, Norton, 1941, 448–449.
13. NEISSER, C. "Katatonia", in: TUKE, D. H. (ed.) *A Dictionary of Psychological Medicine,* London, Churchill, 1892, vol. II, 724–725.
14. ARNDT, E., *op. cit.*
15. HECKER, E. Nekrolog über Kahlbaum. *Monatsschrift für Psychiatrie und Neurologie,* 1899, **5**, 479.
16. MEYER, A. *Collected Papers.* Baltimore, Johns Hopkins Press, 1951, vol. II, 477–486.
17. NEISSER, C. "Karl Ludwing Kahlbaum", in: KIRCHHOFF, T. (ed.) *Deutsche Irrenärzte.* Berlin, Springer, 1924, vol. II, 87–96.
18. JELLIFFE, S. E. Dementia Praecox—An Historical Summary. *New York Medical Journal,* 1910, **91**, 521–531.
19. WENDER, P. H. Dementia praecox: the development of the concept. *Am. J. Psychiatr.,* 1963, **119**, 1143–1151.
20. KRAEPELIN, E. *One Hundred Years of Psychiatry.* Eng. Tr., New York, Citadel, 1962, 116–117.
21. JONG de, H. and BARUK, H. *La catatonie expérimentale par la bulbocapnine: étude physiologique et clinique.* Paris, Masson, 1930.
22. MENNINGER, K. et. al. The unitary concept of mental illness. *Bull. Menninger Clinic,* 1958, **22**, 4–12.
23. GRINKER, R. R. *Toward a Unified Theory of Human Behavior.* New York, Basic Books, 1956. (2nd ed. 1967).
24. LLOPIS, B. *Introduction dialectica a la psicopatologia.* Madrid, Morata, 1970.

PUBLICATIONS OF KARL LUDWIG KAHLBAUM

KAHLBAUM, K. L.: *Entwurf einer Wissenschaftslehre nach der Methode der Naturforschung.* Danzig, 1860.
— *Die Gruppierung der psychischen Krankheiten und die Einteilung der Seelenstörungen.* Danzig, 1863.
— "Die Sinnesdelirien". *Allgemeine Zeitschrift für Psychiatrie,* **23**, 1 (1866).
— "Über Spannungsirresein". Lecture. Ref. *Archiv für Psychiatrie,* **2**, 502 (1870).
— *Klinische Abhandlungen über psychische Krankheiten.* 1. Heft: "Die Katatonie oder das Spannungsirresein". Berlin, 1874.
— *Die klinisch-diagnostischen Gesichtspunkte der Psychopathologie.* Leipzig, 1878.
— "Über zyklisches Irresein". *Irrenfreund,* Nr. 10 (1882).
— "Über jugendliche Nerven- und Gemütskranke und ihre pädagogische Behandlung in der Heilanstalt". *Allgemeine Zeitschrift für Psychiatrie,* **40**, 863 (1884).
— "Über eine klinische Form des moralischen Irreseins". Lecture. Ref. *Allgemeine Zeitschrift für Psychiatrie,* **41**, 711 (1885).
— "Über eine klinische Form des moralischen Irreseins". Lecture. Ref. *Archiv für Psychiatrie,* **16**, 570 (1885).
— "Über Heboidophrenie", *Allgemeine Zeitschrift für Psychiatrie,* **46**, 461 (1890).
— "Über einen Fall von Pseudoparanoia", *Allgemeine Zeitschrift für Psychiatrie,* **49**, 486 (1893).

Introduction

In this monograph I intend to publish a number of findings based on the data collected during my observation of patients in two asylums; the material concerns specialized subjects and consists partly of clinical demonstrations held by me at the East Prussian Provincial Institute for students of the Königsberg University. Although all the hitherto published textbooks of psychiatry condemn as untenable the views according to which these clinical forms of diseases are normally classed as melancholy, mania, etc., the particular treatment of each disease still acknowledges this system; I therefore decided not to refer to any textbooks at all in my lectures and bedside demonstrations but to develop the description of the diseases according to the clinical method, using if possible all the vital expressions of individual patients for diagnostic purposes and for assessing the entire course of the disease. Thus I grouped together the symptoms that were most frequent and often coincided, and by purely empirical classification I obtained groups of diseases which only partly and indirectly coincided with the previous classification; this system was not merely more comprehensible to the listeners, but the diagnostic based on it also enabled me to reconstruct the previous course of the disease from the present state of a patient; moreover, I was able to predict the future development not only in general *quoad vitam* and *valetudinem*, but also in details regarding the various phases of the symptomatic picture—furthermore, with greater reliability than would have been possible on the basis of the previous classification. Although my observations were mostly concluded by then, i.e. more than seven years ago, I was unable to publish them sooner because I had taken over the private observations of persons from quite different social strata, confirmed the reliability of my previous observations and the conclusions drawn from them, and many discussions with colleagues proved to me the extraordinary demonstrability of the new forms of diseases; I therefore no longer hesitate to proceed with the publication.

In the meantime the trend of psychiatric studies has changed and been clarified to a considerable extent. There was a time when any special psychiatric observation was viewed with disapproval if it did not conclude with a thorough anatomical analysis. This anatomicopathological work, undertaken with the most commendable zeal, produced much valuable material but contributed nothing to the basic views on the origin of mental illnesses or on the anatomical basis of their diverse and significant manifestations; the view is now spreading that only comprehensive clinical observation of cases can bring order and clarity into the material by using the method of clinical pathology, and thus prepare ground for greater psychiatric progress with the aid of anatomical data. It has now been recognized that it is futile to search for an anatomy of melancholy or mania, etc., because each of these forms occurs under the most varied relationships and combinations with other states, and they are just as little the expressions of an inner pathological process as the complex of symptoms called fever or the collective name dropsy can in the case of certain somatic diseases be considered to characterize them or to be their particular substratum.

How wrong it inevitably was to expect pathological anatomy alone to reform the obsolete psychiatric framework and to neglect more or less all other ways is proved by the development of other pathological specializations. What improvements in neuropathology occurred when there was as yet no neurohistology, and how well did distinctions and classifications, obtained by physiological and clinical observations, prove themselves in neuropathology even later, when pathological anatomy made several confident strides into the field of neuropathy! I wish to mention, for instance, Morbus basedowii, bulbar paralysis and aphasia. But the clinical method is of great interest for yet another reason: it successfully combats the ever-spreading empty scepticism and idle nihilism that held sway in psychiatry for so long, and it provides a useful support for practical requirements.

The first step in the clinical method was marked in psychiatry by the definition of the so-called *general paralysis of the insane*. The observations of the old somatic school had already emphasized that a number of the psychiatric diseases are accompanied with paralytic symptoms. The subject, until then dismissed as incidental among the *complications of insanity*, has assumed extraordinary importance owing to the clinical definition of a special disorder in which the paralytic phenomena form only a series of symptoms; its significance is such that most additions to the psychiatric literature for many years have been almost exclusively works dealing with this subject. This one clinical form of disorder has all this time remained almost the only object yielding results for the analytical work of pathological anatomy in psychiatry; this seems to prove that research in this domain requires clinical preparatory work ("Propaedeutics"). However, current textbooks treat almost exclusively this psychiatric illness according to the clinical method and only in case of complications; the example it provides of a clinical definition of diseases has not been taken up for constructing similar clinical groups of mental illnesses; it has only served to reconcentrate the observations on somatic complications. It is the French who discovered this first form and who now, almost alone, are making new attempts at further progress in clinical treatment ("folie circulaire")* without allowing themselves to be confused by the somatic-neurological symptom which, of course, is a very pronounced trait of this form. For decades the somatic symptoms of psychoses had been eagerly observed and collected by psychiatrists; nevertheless, it was not the existence of the somatic symptom that endowed this disease with its scientific and practical importance but the clinical method of its definition and description; that the method current in general pathology was used with more dexterity in somatic processes is the reason that just this form of the disease assumed at first such importance for psychiatry. Somatic symptoms and somatic observation of psychiatric diseases have been used repeatedly to discover new paths for general psychopathology or to make individual statements aimed at the general clarification of the psychiatric material. However, mere pathological observation and statistical survey of the incidence of individual somatic symptoms—no matter how interesting in themselves—and their industrious exploitation for more general considerations and uniformity of the specialized pathological material**only lead to rationalistic or merely nominal transformation of the old psychiatric forms without changing definitions, just as the previous psychiatry, which confined itself mostly to changing psychological terminology, merely provided a mass of new synonyms and introduced more and more confusion into the nomenclature. This yielded neither a lasting enrichment of valuable experiences nor a rational psychopathology.

Only a comprehensive and intensive application of the clinical method can enable psychiatry to progress and to increase the understanding of psychopathological processes. Then, the indivudual experiences of casuistic empiricism, accumulated in numerous large hospitals for mental patients (but which are now largely disappearing with the bearer of the experience on account of the differences of nomenclature), will not be lost to psychiatry; on the basis of mutual communication usable material will be gained for later utilization, and individual and general phenomena observed in psychiatric patients will contribute to ever-increasing knowledge.

This scientific analysis of psychological and somatic phenomena will also give wider scope to the anatomical research into psychopathological states and processes and to the anatomical clarification of individual forms of disease; after all, this

---

*JEAN-PIERRE FALRÉT (1794–1870). De la folie circulaire. *Bull. Acad. Méd.,* 1854, **19**, 382.

**For instance, the observation, in itself correct, that in cases of melancholic disorders tonic cramps are more frequent than not gave rise to the idea that melancholy is a kind of tonic cramp of the soul; on the other hand, the agitation of a maniac was compared to clonic cramps, while dementia invited a comparison with paralysis. This neuropathological parallelism gave immediate rise to a reshaping of the three old main forms of psychiatric ilnesses: melancholy was now called psychic tonism, mania psychic clonism and dementia psychic paralysis. But nothing was gained for psychiatry except additional terminology, without the slightest change in the pathological content!

clarification should in all cases be the keystone and touchstone of pathological knowledge.

Entering into even greater detail about the method which I call clinical, I want to point first of all to somatic clinical medicine, which has taught us that rational pathology does not study the disease by itself but studies the patient with all his vital functions, furthermore that no symptomatic phenomenon is considered too trifling, even if it does not seem to refer to the diseased organ; if normal physiology cannot provide an explanation, it is to be studied thoroughly by pathology, possibly split up into further individual phenomena and made the object of attention by being given a new name. Thus in psychiatry, too, all vital manifestations in the insane must be the object of pathological study, and it is right and necessary that somatic processes also be studied and collected according to the rules of clinical semiology and diagnostic technique and with all available scientific means; this is something that the somatic-psychiatric school pointed out and endeavored to achieve decades ago, in opposition to the moralizing theoreticians. Nevertheless, somatic phenomena, especially non-neurological ones, are only of second-rate interest to psychiatric research in most cases; the psychiatric phenomena in the narrower and broader sense—I say in the broader sense because in physiology and pathology it is impossible to draw a clear dividing line between psychiatric and neurological-somatic phenomena—remain the main subject of psychiatric study. Within the psychiatric phenomena this main clinical requirement is repeated: the insane person, in his entirety, all the psychic and neurotic processes, have to be taken into account and studied individually, not in the manner of psychology, where the traditional tendency demands that all phenomena be deduced from a single principle as part of a uniform whole, but by the method of natural science, i.e. as individual natural phenomena, for which the pathologist must create his own physiological analysis if he does not find a ready-made one in physiology. The mistake of deriving all phenomena from one principle may occur in somatic and physiological (materialistic) as well as in philosophical and psychological concepts; for instance, when all psychic phenomena are reduced to the single scheme of the reflex process, it is no more a lasting contribution to science than when the philosophical schools deduced this from the principle of identity or that of polarity, etc. The psychic phenomena have first to be viewed and compiled quite without prejudice, like individual phenomena in other natural sciences, and only when substantial material comes to be available in at least a somewhat different form and in greater abundance than hitherto will it be possible to attempt causal or physiological and anatomical substantiation; only then, when a number of individual phenomena have been subjected to a fundamental analysis, can an attempt be made at a comprehensive comparison and simplification. In this, no other branch of science can be of substantial assistance to psychiatry. Psychiatry itself, following the methods of physiology and the natural sciences, must make a thorough study of the psychic phenomena, and just as some fields of somatic physiology have been treated scientifically and physiologically on the basis of pathology and by pathologists, so, or even more so, is original work by psychiatrists necessary in order that collected material be elaborated scientifically to attain a rich and truly scientific psychology or psychophysiology. It seems to me that here the main shortcoming of the present psychopathology comes to the fore, showing itself as the cause of stagnation in clinical psychiatry. The well-founded discrediting of former psychopathological views and research coincided with the collapse of those presumptuous castles in the air of natural philosophy which could not even hold their own in the realm of the moral sciences, much less be objects of natural science. This led psychiatrists to ignore the psychic aspect of the vital manifestations of insane persons, and precisely the most direct symptoms of the organs most susceptible to disease—for these are the psychiatric symptoms—were not thoroughly studied by psychopathology. This must be remedied immediately, for nothing facilitates clinical observation as much as thorough and accurate symptomatology. However, one should not be deterred by the mass of absolutely necessary minute and detailed work, nor should one hesitate to proceed with the simplest scientific operations, in accordance with the methods applied in the first phases of development in the natural sciences. Beyond the mental processes, listed by present psychology, there is a whole world of psychic details which from the psychological point of view are still terra incognita and can only be discovered by laborious search, although they are contained in the overall psychic phenomena, occur before the eyes of the world at large and can be found scattered as hints in writings where one would least look for them, particularly in works by dramatists and novelists. No one is confronted with these psychic phenomena in their natural analysis so closely and frequently as the psychiatrist, who in a case of illness can observe experimental states provided by nature. Here it is necessary to find one's way in the labyrinth of the manifestations, and there is no better means to this end than the clinical designation, i.e., the nomenclature. This expedient should not be despised although it provides only temporary aid and is already obsolete in some branches. Even the blossom of modern medicine, pathological anatomy, had to resort to this recently on a large scale. In the field of psychic phenomena a richer terminology will be even more necessary to allow for more thorough research.

Thus the detailed observation and more frequent treatment of psychic phenomena in insane persons and the inception of a specialized scientific psychiatric symptomatology are further urgent requirements of clinical psychopathology. It may sound paradoxical but it is a fact that psychopathology, which years ago was censured because of its emphasis on symptoms, did in fact have so symptomatology at all, and in psychiatric textbooks symptomatology was accorded by far the least space. Of course, if psychiatric symptomatology meant, as a psychiatrist of that period once said to me, that the single objects of normal psychology have to be taken only negatively or pathologically changed, and that would provide the psychiatric symptomatology, then it would be better if it remained unwritten. But the psychiatrist has to create, together with the symptomatology, his correct and relevant applied psychology, and in this he has to proceed ruthlessly, depending on whether the most conspicuous phenomenon is important, practically or scientifically, and whether it leads to more far-reaching gains or not.

Upon such thorough observation of the vital phenomena of the patient (the somatic as well as the psychic, and among the psychic the intellectual as well as the affective and ethical, the conscious and voluntary and the unconscious and involuntary), it is obvious from the start that the old names of diseases cannot possibly apply, even temporarily, to what they still designate in practice, although this had been criticized. Predictably, new definitions emerge spontaneously very rapidly, for in the field of natural psychic processes the situation is the same as in other natural fields, where further discoveries have been inevitable once the path has been cleared and smoothed by an initial one. Such a first discovery was the recognition of an entirely novel kind of psychiatric form of disease according to a hitherto unused method of definition, which we may call the clinical method, as opposed to the former methods working according to uniform psychological or unilaterally somatic principles, viz. that of general paralysis of the insane. Another achievement of the new clinical method is definition of the group of diseases designated by me as "juvenile insanity" or "hebephrenia," which Dr. Hecker described specially on the basis of my statement and collection of case histories, some of which he also observed (*Virch. Arch. für path. Anat.* [Virchow Archive for Pathological Anatomy], Vol. 52). A number of other such definitions, of which the first is "catatonia", is to be given special clinical elaboration in these pages.

I am well aware how far my work lags behind what should and can be achieved by the method I have used, which is the method of all clinical medicine; however, I am certain that psychiatry will make decisive progress only along this path, and I therefore feel obliged to publish these partly fragmentary studies to promote the scientific inquiry along these lines.

Concerning the group of diseases first dealt with in this work, viz. catatonia, I wish to point out that I demonstrated it as long as seven years ago in my clinical and theoretical lectures at Königsberg University, when I gave a comprehensive survey at the psychiatric section of the naturalists' assembly at Innsbruck (1868) and at an assembly of the Psychiatrists' Society in Berlin (1871). No special report has been published of either assembly, and it is therefore not surprising that my data on catatonia are very incompletely known and comprehended; this can be deduced by its mention at the psychiatric section of the naturalists' assembly at Leipzig (1872), where it was introduced into the discussion in my absence on the occasion of a lecture by Dr. Arndt on tetany and psychosis.

Görlitz, September 1873 **Dr. Kahlbaum**

1

Preliminary Definitions of Criteria and Medical Case Histories

Even in the early stages of psychopathological studies one fact stood out, namely, that most mental patients also show signs of organic disease which may have a marked effect on their psychic disorder. The evaluation of the relative importance of these organic symptoms is known to have frequently been a bone of contention among the different schools of thought in psychiatry. Some regarded the organic symptoms as chance complications of the correlated mental disorder, whereas others suggested that they displayed elements referable to this disorder. Although the so-called somatic school of nosology seems finally to have gained the upper hand in this dispute, the criteria of the opposing view of the "psychogenetic" school of nosology are still applicable in determining differences and definitions of psychiatric disorders; in spite of the principle to the contrary, somatic complaints were treated as a side issue, to be investigated more thoroughly only if they were likely to be of importance in determining the prognosis and treatment of the psychiatric disorder, or if they were apt to shed some light on the etiology of such disorders in specific cases. They were not regarded of interest in determining the nature of the correlated illness, nor were they used in attempts to define its limits; the only exception to this practice was GPI (General Paralysis of the Insane)—of luetic (syphilitic) etiology.

With respect to this disease, clinical concepts have also changed over the years. At first, the paralytic component was regarded merely as a complication of the correlated illness, but it gradually became clear that the psychiatric disorders involved were present more specifically in association with pathognomonic paralytic phenomena typical only of this disease, and that there was a closer connection between the progress of psychic phenomena and somatic components. The somatic components also seemed to be specific to this disease alone. Later it transpired that

GPI can occur clinically without delusions of grandeur, and at the same time it emerged that the paralytic components were identical with those found in Tabes dorsalis, both forms having their etiology in degeneration of the posterior columns of gray matter in the spinal cord. Still more recently there have been attempts to show that in the past the entire complex clinical picture of GPI had included various differing clinical manifestations lumped together under one heading; there seems to have been some return to the original hypothesis that, at least for some of the cases with this disease, the paralytic manifestations can be regarded only as a complication of the psychiatric disorder itself. It must be admitted, though, that irrespective of the final evaluation of this relationship, the paralytic component of the disease in cerebrovascular syphilis is from the pathological point of view of much greater significance than any somatic disturbance in most other forms of mental illness; it is precisely because of this that GPI presents an excellent opportunity for a study of somatic disorders and of the role they play in the clinical pattern in psychiatric disorders.

In this work I will attempt to describe a disease pattern which has somatic components, with particular involvement of the musculature; they occur as often here as in GPI, and go along with certain psychic manifestations of the disease; in this particular mental disorder they also play an important part in the form taken by the entire process of the disease.

This illness is closely related to the mental disorder usually termed atonic melancholia ("melancholia attonita"); it was usually regarded as a separate disease entity, although its occurrence in the primary form is extremely rare. It generally constitutes a stage in the more commonly known melancholic illness or in most cases following melancholia (depression) with a subsequent manic phase; atonic melancholia (or depression) may thus be regarded as the third phase of the disease. If recovery from this stage fails to take place, there may be a deterioration into a terminal, fourth, stage—terminal dementia. The course of this condition seems to corroborate the observations of Guislain, Zeller, and Griesinger, who maintained that mental illness may run a course exhibiting different stages which present different signs and symptoms, so that it is incorrect to regard simple melancholia, manic states, or the form known as atonic melancholia each as a distinct and separate disease entity.

The typical signs of the condition termed atonic melancholia may be described as a state in which the patient remains entirely motionless, without speaking, and with a rigid, masklike facies, the eyes focused at a distance; he seems devoid of any will to move or react to any stimuli; there may be a fully developed "waxen" flexibility, as in cataleptic states, or only indications, distinct, nevertheless, of this striking phenomenon. The general impression conveyed by such patients is one of profound mental anguish, or an immobility induced by severe mental shock; it has been classified either among the states of depression (which explains the term atonic melancholia) or among the conditions of feeble-mindedness (stupor or dementia stupida); others have regarded it as a combination of the two (Baillarger's "mélancholie avec stupeur"). Once the clinical signs are manifest, they tend to persist, although in some patients they appear for relatively short periods and then tend to recur. The symptoms are at times not as strikingly severe as those described above, and when these are lacking it is difficult to assess the condition of the patient in its true context. The obvious association of this illness with other signs of disease, and its constant occurrence with certain somatic (particularly muscular) disorders, have been more or less ignored.

If the cases of this particular mental illness, which in its course shows overt signs of atonic melancholia—for brevity called here atonicity—are subjected to a thorough clinical investigation, it will be noted that in many patients the disorder may manifest itself in various clinical signs, such as epileptiform seizures or allied spastic conditions which appear intermittently; subsequently the intervals between spastic attacks become less frequent. In the atonic stage of the disease they are most striking and take the form of waxen atonicity or flexibility; lingering signs of this condition may still be evident in the stage of terminal dementia. These interesting somatic features are as unique in the diagnosis of this particular illness as are the somatic components of general paralysis of the insane, in the presence or absence of delusions of grandeur, and they are certainly of equal importance. In addition, the clinical features of atonic melancholia also include certain somatic, but in particular psychic, elements. They may be described as a state of exaltation of a peculiar type, a certain pathos-filled "ecstasy"; this entrains a compulsion to talk in oratorical style which, together with other signs and the atonicity described, seems to be typical of the disease.

Clinically, therefore, it may be said that this disease has certain features which may be regarded as a pattern similar to the present in general paralysis of the insane, with or without delusions of grandeur. In some aspects, such as the clinical course marked by the passage through various phases of distinct mental states and the significant association with muscular disorders, the one is analogous to the other. In other respects, on the other hand, concerning for instance the patterns of muscular and psychic disorders and the prognosis of the illness (as will be emphasized later), the illness under discussion contrasts fundamentally from the other. Atonic melancholia is not merely of general and clinical interest; its frequency of occurrence and the anthropological factors involved place its importance on a wider scale.

1. Case history

Benjamin L.* (case report by Chief Physician Dr. Hammer, Dr. Munch, and Municipal Medical Officer in Königsberg, Prussia), 27 years old, country-school teacher,

---

*The names of patients have been changed throughout.

son of a farmer; having studied in a country school under a particularly capable teacher, first learnt the saddlery (leather workshop) trade, and after working for eighteen months as an apprentice, decided to go in for teaching. Studied with a teacher for one year, and after passing the required examination, was appointed on an interim basis as assistant to the head teacher at a country school; he taught here for 4 years until he fell ill.

Psychiatric data. Intellectual abilities appear average; apparently has a "choleric" temperament, shows little emotional independence; otherwise no psychological disorders (no tendencies to abnormal behavior, no alcoholism, etc.). Physical development and clinical findings normal.

There were no known illnesses in his past history.

Some time before the actual symptoms of the disease became evident, the patient began to suffer moods of depression, which were at first masked and alternated with violent affective reactions; later the moods became more clearly manifest. During states of particular irritability, he was often induced to behave unfairly to his pupils, and was frequently reprimanded on this account by the authorities. As the state of melancholia progressed, the patient's mental acuity deteriorated; this state was accompanied with choreiform facial "tics," at first seemingly partly voluntary, but later entirely involuntary; these tics went together with jerking spastic movements of the extremities; at first the patient was able to control or modify these movements, but later he lost control completely. At this point he was admitted to a hospital (Krankenhaus der Barmherzigkeit) in Königsberg.

Now follows the hospital medical report: B's illness consists of spastic contractions of the facial and cervical musculature, as well as of other groups of muscles (extremities); no somatic condition has been found to explain these phenomena. The following behavioral aberrations have been noted: The patient would often stand alone and upright in a corner for periods of about half an hour at a time, gesticulating extravagantly with his arms; at night he tended to wander about on his own in the dark house, etc.

The Municipal Medical Officer, Dr. Janert, continues the case history: Since his admission to hospital, the patient has been living in an isolated world of his own, is almost entirely noncommunicative, and most of the time appears deep in thought. He shows no interest in any mental or physical activity; he has a slouching posture, halting gait, and all his movements show lassitude; his head is bowed, his eyes downcast, their expression hesitant and timid; his speech is slow, with emphasis on each phrase, and when reading aloud, full of pathos; he evinces no interest in his past occupation or in his physical well-being; he is not concerned about his future and is largely apathetic to what goes on around him. He is attentive to questions directed to him, and his memory is unimpaired; he is capable of providing exact information concerning personal relationships, yet each attempt to induce him to formulate continuous thoughts or to synthesize more complicated thought processes triggers a reaction consisting of the choreiform muscle activity described above. There is also an unmistakable impairment of intelligence and his powers of self control are at times absent, not only with respect to involuntary muscle movements. Left to himself, he persists in a state of aimless introspection, shows no signs of being aware of his surroundings or of purpose-directed mental activity, and is incapable of directing or controlling his mental wanderings. Hallucinations or states of delusion of grandeur seem to be absent. The course of the illness is progressive, without remissions. There seem as yet to be no signs of behavior dangerous to other, but the fear of this possibility remains.

Etiology. No hereditary factors are present. The main etiological factor seems to be weakening of the nervous system due to onanism; this assumption is borne out to some extent by the patient's downcast, hesitant gaze, his sallow complexion, and his entire confidence-lacking demeanor.

In the East Prussian Institute at Allenberg. Admitted 21 September 1861. Patient's height 5'6", somewhat underweight, but seems sturdy, body build normal. Hair brown; eyes brown; on examination, pulse somewhat slow and weak. The patient is completely motionless; sits or stands stiffly on one spot. Eyes open, pupils equal and of normal size. Gaze fixed, mouth somewhat open, its left corner a little higher, otherwise no facial assymetry; facial musculature flaccid, nose pointed. Neck slightly extended backwards, arms hanging loosely at the sides. B. fails to answer any questions put to him or to talk while being examined. He does not budge from one spot; when raised he remains standing, if pushed or induced to change his position he reacts slowly, showing some resistance. Reacts only with a grimace to needlepricks on hands and feet; allows the introduction of a seton under the skin of the neck without displaying a marked muscle pain reflex. Does not extend his tongue. Must be led to the table to eat; when ordered to take a spoon in his hand, does so after hesitating for some time; is eventually able to bring the spoon to his mouth; eats very little. Has to be dressed and undressed. At certain intervals (several times a day every few days) has attacks of muscle spasms involving the arms and corners of the mouth. Has very severe constipation.

The patient remained in the condition described for many months. Only the following temporary changes were registered from time to time: it was occasionally possible to encourage him to show greater awareness of his surroundings. Gradually he was induced to leave his bed voluntarily and to dress and undress without aid. In his sitting posture he had for long periods resembled the prototypes of the giant Egyptian stone statues: a stiff posture with the upper half of the body held rigid for hours or even days, the forearms resting on the thighs, his eyes staring unwaveringly in front of him. The expression he wore could not be described as showing signs of mental stress; it rather seemed devoid of feeling and detached. When observed for longer periods, he evinced slight movement, a contortion of the facial muscles indicating displeasure. At times he sagged to the left side and remained sitting with the torso partly bent. At other times he was seen to bend his head to the left, and on one occasion to the right, but these postures were witnessed more rarely. At times he directed his gaze partly upward for hours on end. He was sometimes observed with his eyes closed; upon an attempt to open them, the eyelid muscles showed a prolonged tremor. Extremities emaciated; passive movements were easily carried out; if placed in any particular position, the limbs remained thus for some length of time, but the patient gradually resumed his original posture. Sensory response was somewhat reduced over the entire body surface. Pricking with a needle almost always elicited a response, even if slight. Events taking place in the room had no effect on him; in time it was possible to persuade him to carry out instructions directing him to participate in the communal meals, to go to sleep, etc. For a long time he still had to be reminded to carry out these various routine tasks. He also remained standing at the table long after prayers were over, until the orderly pressed him to sit down. With few exceptions, he did not refuse food, but at first had to be persuaded to eat with the aid of others. His appetite and his excretory functions gradually improved. His feet were often swollen.

A seton was introduced under the skin of the neck. It was kept in place for about 5 weeks, without leading to any definite improvement in his condition. During treatment with phosphorylated ether for a period of six months, the patient became somewhat more alert. He was mentally fit to the degree that he was able to partake in exercises, to remember his daily chores without being prompted, and to rise voluntarily and approach the physician during the latter's ward round, etc.

After about nine months an incident occurred in which he showed an unusual display of feeling. He embraced the chief medical orderly, laughing and weeping, and walked about in the corridor. This burst of energy was not repeated; another phase of alertness to his surroundings took place several months after this incident, and after having been 16 months in the institute he began to talk and to write. To begin with he spoke only a few words, but was able at the same time to write a fairly long and detailed letter home. He was also persuaded to copy text, to read aloud, and later even to participate in classes and in light physical exercise. His facial expression became only slightly more animated; his movements remained slow and persisted in seeming unrelaxed and stiff. He still had to be reminded frequently to perform routine movements. He undertook no action on his own initiative.

During the following two years spent at the institute, there was little change in his condition. He was usually reluctant to speak, and when he did, he often lapsed into complete silence or limited his vocabulary to a whispered "yes" or "no." When asked whether it was difficult for him to speak, he would reply: "I cannot tell you myself." In fact, although his speech was usually slow and monosyllabic, he was able on rare occasions, when in an alert mood, to speak loudly and at length. There were times when he seemed laconic and reluctant to speak at all to the physicians examining him, but spoke quite animatedly to the orderly who accompanied him on his walks. His conscious being, as far as one could ascertain from the little he spoke, was beset by a constant feeling of insecurity, often accompanied with fear or depressive fantasies which ruled him entirely and which made him feel that "he must not . . . "; a typical conversation with him would proceed as follows: "Do you feel well?"—"Yes, I think so"—Did he feel he was doing his utmost to get well, such as following instructions to exercise?—"Yes."—Had he taken his prescribed walk that day?—"I will, if I am allowed to do so."—Had anyone forbidden him to do certain things?—No answer.—Had anyone told him that he is forbidden to do cetain things?—"No one has said so, but I feel as if I am forbidden to do things."— When the suggestion was put to him to stand up each morning during the physicians' round and to approach them, and he failed to follow this through, he said: "I am not permitted to do so, it is not fitting for me to do this." Later, when he joined working-class patients in gardening activities, he had an uncontrollable fear of being beaten to death. At another stage, the priest attached to the institute took particular interest in him and helped him during classes held there; the patient accused the priest of showing hostility toward him, claiming: "You have got your knife into me. You do not question the others as you do me, I must always be the one to know everything. I don't know what you mean, Reverend, by persisting in questioning me. After all, I am mentally ill. Send me out of here, and then I will know; there are so many learned gentlemen here, ask them about it." It could be said that his performance at classes held at the institute indicated a definite deterioration in intelligence, both in depth as well as in the scope of his mental capacities. His ability to grasp problems and his memory, including recollection of past events and subjects learnt in previous years, were impaired. At the same time one had the impression that the mental processes were not impaired so much as repressed, as if "paralyzed." It must be remembered that the patient's mental activity had undergone progressive deterioration. His mood was mainly one of indifference; sometimes he laughed to himself. He hardly ever wept. Only rarely did his facial expression denote suffering. The states of fear mentioned earlier seemed to have no effect on his usual frame of mind.

He provided no information on reasons for his state of mind; at times he expressed himself well in matters pertaining to his family; he was also able to show more and more interest in details concerning home life during his father's visits. The pattern of his physical activities remained on the whole unaltered, with the same monotonous, slow, awkward and stiff behavior. During the last two years at the institute there had been no convulsive disorders. Sensory perception had returned to normal. After more than three years in the institute, he was discharged and sent home for lack of room there.

An analysis of this patient's course of illness indicates that he first went through a prodromal stage of melancholia or depression, followed by a stage marked by impairment of general mental activity; this state may persist for a long time without actually passing into a state of total dementia, but it comes close to it. This state of mental deterioration is accompanied with convulsive attacks involving the entire muscular system; they initially take the form of choreiform seizures, which at times may be continuous; later they occur in a milder form of more localized convulsions. In the periods free of convulsions there may be partial contractures of muscles or increased flexibility; another phenomenon observed was one of a peculiar mechanism which hinders the patient in carrying out voluntary muscular activity or in maintaining muscle tone. Sensory perception is reduced, but recovers even before the disorders in voluntary muscle innervation and other neurological signs disappear. Other distinct somatic components are the lack of appetite and the absence of tonus of the intestinal musculature and of vascular tonus in the extremities (with appearance of edema).

2. Case history

Julius G. (case reported by Dr. Atzpodien and District Health Officer Dr. Klokowin in Tilsit), 33 years old, a peasant; his mother and one sister had suffered temporary mental illness. Grew up in the country, worked on his father's farm; had recently had a love affair which ended in the spring of 1856 because of unfaithfulness on the girl's part. G. was good-natured, of average intelligence and capacity for a normal life. Physically well developed; showed some sensitivity and changeability of mood during certain climatic changes. Was always in good health.

Psychiatric data. Following the termination of his love affair, G. became depressed; he was often reluctant to talk or to participate in various activities; this state became even more marked when the girl married one year after discontinuing their relationship (in May 1857). On St. John's Day [midsummer's day], a syphilitic infection in the secondary stage was diagnosed. He had apparently been advised by a physician to have sexual relations with another woman in order to get over his disappointment. After this episode, his moods of depression became constant. There was some improvement at the beginning of the following year. But subsequently he began to have convulsive seizures, which occurred several times a day; they consisted partly in muscular twitchings in the face and extremities and partly in more severe tonic contractions of the back muscles; the extent of his awareness fluctuated between full and partial. At the beginning of May there was a further psychic deterioration. Again he avoided contact with people, and during a visit from his aunt, instead of participating with the others in the event, he retired to bed and stayed there. He lay in bed without interest in his surroundings, his eyes shut; he refused to reply when addressed, or even to speak at all. Sympathetic, friendly and comforting words of encouragement were of no avail. Admonishment also failed to alter his attitude, but when severely reprimanded, he at least sometimes reacted with a certain display of activity (such as getting out of bed, putting on his jacket, etc.). During examination by a physician there was no change in his behavior: his eyes could be opened only by force and he could not be induced to utter a single word. His facial expression was melancholy and anguished; when at rest his breathing was slow and regular, but it quickened and became somewhat uneven with a sighing quality during a medical examination. No abnormalities were found upon examination of the chest and lower parts of the body. The urine had a reddish tinge. Bowel movements were irregular, infrequent, the stools hard. His appetite varied; on the whole he ate adequately, but he refused to eat anything served him while someone else was present; he also had the peculiar habit of leaving some food even if given minimal quantities. Muscular development average. Pulse regular. Perspired a great deal. Slept a lot by day and at night. He often had urinary incontinence, but for bowel movements he did make use of the chamber pot placed next to him. At a later date (29 June) the physician once entered the room without speaking, and remained seated at G.'s bedside for 15 minutes without uttering a word. The patient's eyes were shut; he then began to breathe less regularly and to sigh; finally he opened his eyes, but closed them immediately on noticing the doctor. It was not possible to induce him to utter a word. G. showed a persistent tendency to perspire. At that time his bowel movements became more regular and his urine less reddish. At times he would get out of bed. Date: 22 August. Bleeding of gums and lips, the latter covered with little scabs. At attempts to be led into the main room, did not open his eyes; when support was withdrawn, he did not fall, but staggered to his bed with his eyes shut. Excessive sweating ceased. There were no other changes in his condition.

G. was admitted to the institute at Allenberg on 28 December 1863. He spent the first three months there in an unchanging state of inactivity. He remained lying prone in his bed, gave no answer to questions put to him, and kept his eyes constantly closed. They could be opened only by force, whereupon he immediately shut them again. He showed some resistance to attempts to lift or raise him, but allowed himself to be helped out of bed and to be undressed. Any posture he was made to assume he tended to maintain for prolonged periods. As in states of catalepsy, here too it was possible to place the patient's extremities in the most extravagant positions; these he maintained for a long time and only gradually changed, to return to his original passive position. His musculature was very weak, and his state of nutrition very poor. There was no noticeable contraction and shortening of the muscles involved in extension or flexion. At times he would get up of his own volition to use the toilet facilities, but more often he would pass urine in bed. Bowel movements occurred at very rare intervals. His appetite was poor. G. ate only when alone in his room. Accepted medicines proffered. If a spoon was placed in his hand, he took it, but soon put it back. When induced to attempt some steps, he moved forward slowly, leaning to the right a little, and extended his right leg stiffly. Sensory response was greatly reduced over the entire body. Reaction to needle-pricking was absent most of the time. Feet showed edema. A seton inserted during the first period of his stay at the institute was removed in the middle of March.

Toward the end of March there was a change in one aspect of the patient's behavior. Instead of his absolute refusal to speak, he now began to talk incessantly; the scope of his conversation was limited to a few monotonous phrases pertaining to the subjects of love and religious fantasies. For example, one day he repeated the words: "Love is God, Love, Love is God, Love is God." And on another day: "God in God, God, God in God, God in Love, God, God, God, God in Love," etc. Or: "God-Love-God, we thank You: Father, I am Your child; God, Love, God," and so on. Or: "You triple Great God, you triple Great God." On some days he would add short phrases to these repetitions, such as "Is it so?" or "I say," "really." At times the words were spoken softly, on other occasions they were shouted in a vociferous outburst. He continued his incessant talking into the night, but less loudly. If someone placed a hand on his forehead, he fell to uttering the same or similar words in a whisper. At itmes he would alternate between loud and whispered repetitions of a series of words. While doing this he usually lay quite flat on his back, or with the upper part of the body partly raised and head bent stiffly back. Sometimes he enunciated these words with an effort through his teeth, or tended break down single words slowly and painfully syllable by syllable, as if forced to utter them against his will. There were also times when his mouth and eye muscles contracted in cramplike distortion while speaking. He soon became extremely hoarse, and spoke very softly for a long time, with intermittent shouting. His talking ceased between 19 May and 2 June, but then again recommenced in the former manner. This condition persisted, with brief interruptions, almost up to his death, which occurred on 21 August. When he became physically very weak, his voice changed to a sort of grunt or wheeze, finally to become a soft moan. At the beginning of April he had contracted fever and a mild cough. This condition developed into acute tuberculosis of the right lung, which led to his death.

In analyzing the details of the course of the disease in this patient, we note that here again the illness had commenced with a protracted and progressive depression; this condition seemed to improve a little after one year, but recurred and progressed to a strange state of refusal to speak and of inactivity which lasted over a period of 16 months. It is difficult to say whether this state can be denoted as a melancholic condition or "melancholia" proper. In the later phases of the illness there was a marked impairment of mental acuity and predominant irritability and confusion verging on dementia. Later still, the patient became intensely preoccupied with religious fantasies, which dominated the clinical picture together with the major symptom of incessant talking consisting of automatic repetition of the same words or sentences.

The physical symptoms included convulsive seizures of varying form on the one day, followed by the same waxen flexibility or atonicity, which was particularly marked in this case. The patient also had a tendency to spasm-like attacks of the eye and oral musculature during attempts to speak. There were no motor disorders such as pareses, but it should be noted that he sometimes tended to keep the upper part of his body bent to one side and to drag his leg stiffly on the same side. Sensory loss was severe. Here, too, there was some measure of refusal to eat and severe malnutrition.

3. Case history

Baroness Minna von B. (data obtained from relatives), 45 years old. Described as a woman of a particularly mild-mannered and kindly disposition, but at the same time as being noticeably easily irritated and highly strung. Good mother and busy housewife. Physically well developed, robustly healthy as a young girl; later she suffered a great deal from weak nerves and pains. Three normal deliveries over a period of 3 years; she did not breast-feed her children. The third delivery (1839) was accompanied with marked loss of blood, and she subsequently suffered from chronic anemia. In 1850 she had a severe cholera infection; she contracted the disease in a region said to be entirely free of it, solely as a result of her receiving the information that in a district 20 miles distant from her home, her father, sister and brother-in-law had succumbed to cholera.

Psychiatric data. The nervous disorders now increased greatly in intensity, although the patient underwent various cures at different freshwater and other spas; the disorders were associated with very obvious idiosyncrasies, strange behavior and frequently occurring states of nervous excitation. In 1856 she decided with tremendous conviction that the only treatment which would help her was a cold-water cure; the same winter, she proceeded to undergo a rigorous cold-water cure on an intensive scale. She thus acquired physical tolerance to cold, and after this course, remained a fanatic adherent of cold-water cures, to an extent which bordered on pathological obsession; however, she never actually recovered from her ailments or ceased to complain of them. In 1861, while she was going through menopause, she became convinced that she had been poisoned by matches left at her bedside. She complained of a metallic taste in her mouth and developed an aversion to metals. Even before she had been preoccupied with religious ideas and practices, but now she claimed to be in direct contact with the Almighty. There were frequent outbursts of temper and anger, which she later attempted to atone for in the most tender and loving manner. She maintained that no physician could evaluate the nature of her ills, and that only she herself, with the aid of the heavenly powers, would succeed in obtaining some relief from her physical suffering. At that time she began to have convulsivelike disorders, actual cramps in her feet, later involving the arms and jaw muscles; they were accompanied with a sound resembling the ticking of a clock, which was audible in her mouth. Later she had fits of weeping and laughing.

In 1866, during the war, she became extremely agitated; she imagined she saw the coffin of her son who was on active service at the time, and had an attack of overt mania. This went along with a compulsion to destroy objects around her and uncontrollable dementia. She had to be admitted to an institution. Upon admission, she entered a state of complete apathy which persisted until spring 1867 and during which she was said to have presented "a pitiful appearance."

Up to July 1868 she underwent alternate periods of nervous excitation, in part induced by visits from her relatives, and states of complete apathy. While her mental state was lucid up to a point, her behavior was in many ways abnormal, particularly since she was prone to use words which she made up herself; she employed these to a greater degree when in a state of increased excitation, when various absurdities in her behavior became more evident. Her main complaint was that she was constantly aware of noise made by machinery, which plagued her incessantly and ordered her to do various things. It was in this condition that she came to me for treatment.

She was tall, imposing, and powerfully built, with strong features and a kindly expression; her overall behavior gave the impression of premature aging. Her clinical progress could be separated into three main phases. The first was expressed by her sitting in an immobile position, her limbs folded close to her body, cowering. She refused to answer any question put to her; showed some resistance to attempts to move her limbs passively, evinced a slight degree of increasing flexibility of the limbs. Sensory perception was fairly well preserved. The second phase expressed itself in marked talkativeness; she talked to herself or to her surroundings and conjured up reminiscences which were in part fairly coherent and sensible; on the other hand, she tended to veer off into fantasies which were sometimes puerile or at any rate revealed an illogical train of thought and a certain haughtiness, with unrealistic chatter; in her talk she revealed marked lascivious sensuality which seemed to play a part in her fantasies. At times she had definite hallucinations concerning persons whom she insisted were present. She had a compulsion to alter the names of people around her; some of these were names from her previous circle of acquaintances and home surroundings and some were names she had invented. She spoke of herself in the second person, e.g. she might say "shake hands with the doctor" or "do not give him your hand now," "bid him goodbye," etc. At times she spoke as if reciting a lesson learned by heart and did not allow interruption; there were also times at which it was possible to carry on a sensible conversation with her. Her moods changed; most of the time she seemed indifferent, but sometimes she wept bitterly or was playfully jocular. Her attitude to people around her changed too—according to her mood or personal feelings she could be friendly, or unfriendly to a degree which induced her to use abusive language or even to resort to physical force to emphasize her hostility. One of her letters from this period went as follows: "You will receive 100 ducats and 100 Reichsthaler, and with this the payment is settled. Frau von Gladitsch must receive this, and it must be done. Adolphine will also receive this amount, and so will Puppsi, as well as Celestine. Doctor Nimrod or Baron de Nimrod will also receive 100 ducats and 100 Reichsthaler, and Louise also gets 200 ducats and 200 Reichsthaler. Mr. Immerwahr will receive 500 ducats and no more. Frau von Gledisch will also receive another 500 ducats, for the time being no more, because an Empress and an Emperor Fritz B. can settle this payment, because he himself is rich besides your and his family. Baroness B., who in fact is Empress of the entire world, and the daughter and sister-in-law of the Emperor Fritz and your husband, Baron B., and the young Baron Edwin B., actually Emperor of the world, can settle payments and give whatever she wants to whomever she wishes. Her child and her very modest husband want to grant your wishes, Empress of the entire world, whether they believe me or not, since Faith makes one blessed. Thus says Fritz Baron von B. and Edwin Baron von B., and the old gentleman Emperor von B."

At first she took great care to maintain order and cleanliness, but later she often became slovenly and careless of hygiene. She also frequently showed a marked disregard for "decent" behavior; the most obviously erratic actions expressed themselves in a frequent impulse to undress and to walk about only scantily clad. On one occasion she persistently tore out the hairs on her head one by one, and only forcible preventive action stopped her from becoming entirely bald. She was also prone to tear her clothes into shreds. She explained all her actions as being either through God's command or by her own will. At times she was able to occupy herself usefully with simple handicraft. The third phase of her illness, a state between the two extremes described and the one which was by far the most frequently occurring phase, was one during which she sat quietly on the couch, constantly twisting a garment in her hands, and gave curt answers to questions put to her. This habit of twisting a piece of clothing into a sausage-shape had become such a stereotyped activity that the female orderlies attending to her appropriately called it "sausage-making" (würsteln); "the Baroness is making sausages" was a frequent comment. She persisted in this activity so tirelessly and irresistibly, sometimes even at night while half asleep, that it could be regarded almost as a complex type of convulsive or spastic muscle activity.

Again in this case, analysis of the course of the disease reveals an initial state of melancholic depression, which in this patient was actually marked by a hysterical-hypochondriac component which persisted for a long time. During this period there were incidents of repeated convulsions, taking various forms—tonic, functional (uncontrollable laughing and weeping fits), etc. This phase was followed by one of frenzied manic manifestations, passing after a short period to an atonic state, interrupted at intervals by the manic phase. Finally the patient revealed a severe degree of dementia, persisting to date, which was frequently interrupted by short episodes of atonicity or mania. As to the general psychic state of the patient, we can observe how the initially purely "melancholic" state gradually acquired more and more elements of opposing disorders, and finally became entirely submerged. Her normal mental "apparatus" was replaced entirely with a series of distorted concepts, superimposed on a severely disturbed self-awareness; she was able, by means of hallucinations, even to arrive at the concept of direct personal contact with God, and in her later stages, at the idea of being Empress of the entire world. In the final stages the patient's intelligence reverted to a state of puerility. Some aspects of the course of illness are of particular interest, such as the predominance of religious fantasies, the peculiar tendency to refer to herself in the second person, and also the alternation between states of stubborn refusal to speak, which persisted for varying periods, with states in which the patient was overly talkative, repeating certain phrases monotonously and compulsively, even setting these repetitive phrases down in writing. These psychic symptoms were associated with somatic disorders consisting of various convulsive states occurring during the transition from the first to the second stage of the illness; there were also subsequent cataleptiform incidents in the atonic stage. Finally, during the stage of dementia, there were alternating states of peculiar stereotypically performed movements, such as the "sausage-making," and the tightly flexed and contracted posture of the folded limbs.

Several other examples of such cases will be described now only in the form of a resumé.

4. Summary of case history

Adolphine M. (data provided by Dr. Hartoch and District Medical officer Dr. Reichel in M.), 29 years old. Teacher. Eminently suited and well qualified for her job. Physically well built but with a somewhat weak constitution. In the spring of 1858 had an attack of mania which lasted 8 days; no recurrences. August 1863, after a short prodromal stage of physical discomfort, had another manic attack, with predominant compulsion to talk at length; refused food during the 8 days of the attack. This was followed by alternating periods of quiet behavior and relapses into states marked by excessive talkativeness and violent temper tantrums, plus a tendency to do everything the wrong way, although at times she seemed to behave in a perfectly normal manner. In April 1864 was admitted to the institute. For 2 months she seemed to behave sensibly, but did not admit to having had a psychically pathological attack; at the same time she had a somewhat hysterically exaggerated feeling of being ill. At the beginning of July she fell into a state of depressive agitation, with a display of theatrically pathetic behavior; direct and indirect auditory and tactile hallucinations. From 25 July at times had severe atonicity states, i.e., unnaturally stiff posture, inability to move, a need to assume a cowering posture and to remain in a state with contracted muscles for some time; in some measure she had a lack of perception or inability to react to sensory stimuli or to psychic impressions; at times she remained entirely mute, refused food, and became slovenly in personal hygiene. Up to April of the following year her condition deteriorated to such an extreme degree as is seen only in patients who have reached a stage of incurable dementia. She then received a letter from home and reacted with a state of exaltation, but also with a tendency again to do everything wrong. This was followed by apathy, during which she was obsessed with the activity of rubbing all hair off her head. At times she again seemed in a state of excitation. In November she had convulsions involving all the muscles of the extremities—the attack occurred without her uttering a word. 5 November: Tetanic contractions of seemingly all the muscles of the extremities and head region. Did not speak, and when persuaded to talk, shook her head stiffly in the negative and pointed to her mouth and larynx with tightly closed fist and extended finger. Medical examination which followed, as far as was possible at the moment, indicated no changes except for an extraordinary lack of reaction of the pharyngeal mucosa. She then had a mild trismus. On 6 November she relapsed into her previous behavior pattern. A state of apathy prevailed, and she showed an obsessive need to undress. Her nutritional state was very poor because of her refusal to eat; she usually gave an impression of extreme idiocy. In April she became more active, and this state was associated with an obsessive need to abuse everything; at times she talked loudly and incessantly ("verbal diarrhea," as one young colleague accurately described it). This state increased in severity to full-blown mania. Alternations between apathy and manic outbursts persisted until February 1869. At this point the patient's condition improved quite abruptly; she calmed down, and her behavior became consistently more normal and regular. In May it was possible to discharge her in a satisfactory state of health. Although she had no clear concept of the abnormal stages of her illnes, she seemed on the whole to have remained healthy.

5. Summary of case history

Michael G. (data provided by Dr. Steiner and District Health Officer Dr. Beeck, in Pr. Holland). $20\frac{1}{4}$ years old. Rural farm laborer. At the age of 15 years (1855), had an attack of mania 14 days after having worked at a particularly arduous task. In the summers of 1858 and 1859 he had short attacks of temporary insanity. In May 1860 again fell ill after an episode of bloodletting, which he had undergone to cure some undefined ailment described as "confusion in the head," and epistaxis. He then suffered hallucinations of seeing the Devil. Severe attack of violent mania, with remissions and quiet demeanor but confusion still present, persisting until July. Was admitted to the institute in a state akin to catatonia but able to talk.

Minor tendency to somnambulism. Then, on 6 August (during my absence at the time, reported on by my replacement Dr. Riemer) the following details are given: "Since the beginning of August, the patient has had convulsive-type fits, during which isolated groups of muscles seem to be involved consistently. He finds it difficult to walk or to move his arms. His facial musculature is contorted most of the time. It also seems that he had a general convulsive attack involving all limbs. For several days has had epistaxis. Eight leeches were placed. 7 August—holds body in peculiar positions. Either fails to reply to questions, or talks complete nonsense. Remedy: Cupr. Sulph. ammon. 0.25 g, with increase in dosage. 8 August— has had nocturnal urinary incontinence for several nights. 14 August—patient is now calmer. Irritability of motor innervation now reduced, does not have spastic-convulsive tendencies. 24 August—cuprum treatment discontinued. 28 August— the old complaint has recurred." 10 September—repeated manic manifestations. October—severe apathy with some rigidity and complete silence. April 1861— physically and psychically shows signs of increased activity. He was discharged as cured in August.

6. Summary of case history

Adolph L. (data provided by District Health Officer Dr. Kob in L.), 24 years old. Apprentice to pharmacist. Has quite good mental capabilities. Practiced onanism during three years at puberty. In 1862, toward the end of his apprenticeship, he exhibited outstandingly stubborn and sinister characteristics. Although he showed some confusion during the examination, he was appointed assistant pharmacist. 1863—made many mistakes in his job as assistant pharmacist, reluctant to work and defiant. When sent home to his father, he lapsed into insanity. He then became apathetic and used coarse language. Had hallucinations of seeing or hearing the Devil; attacks of uncontrollable rage. Tendency to hold objects in a vice-like grip. Could not be persuaded to use knife and spoon while eating. 1864—1 February. Admitted to the institute. Advanced state of dementia, with apathy and rigidity of the body; at first he was totally mute, later only had periods of refusal to speak; laconic speech persisted; showed lack of cleanliness; his head was bent far forward and held in a rigid manner, the eyes persistently closed, and kept tightly shut. Evinced peculiar movements of the mouth (as during peculiar taste and smell perception), lips tightly pursed or pulled out in a snoutlike expression for long periods ("snout-spasm"). Here, as at home, ate without use of knife or spoon, but insisted stubbornly on drinking soup from the plate; even when eating meat, was prone to avoid the use of his fingers. Showed striking peculiarities of body posture at rest and particularly during movement (when he could be induced to be brought out of his passive behavior). Most often he stood in an isolated corner, both arms pressed against his chest, one hand on his face, the other supporting his elbow. When sitting down, his arms were tightly pressed to his sides. His head was bent forward, and could be raised only with difficulty. While walking, he bent his knees even as he raised them and made the step down with the lateral part of the balls of his feet first. At times it seemed that he would have liked to walk but was unable to commence doing so. Once walking, though, he was able to propel himself forward with a fair speed in spite of the peculiar positioning of his legs and feet. Sensory perception was somewhat reduced, but not overly suppressed. In spite of various attempts to improve his condition by medical preparations, schooling, gymnastics, etc., which he was willing to undertake, there was little change in his condition, and in fact he continued to present a clinical picture of apathy with rigidity and atonicity of a moderate degree.

The case histories described above, to which I could add a considerable number of similar ones, have one important common feature, i.e. the occurrence of definite convulsive fits, sometimes of a general nature, in other cases of only tonic or partly tonic types; these fits or seizures may occur on one occasion only or be repetitive; they may in some instances, even after their cessation, leave residual abnormal changes in the locomotor functions, which may appear in the form of semitonic spastic conditions or incomplete contractures of the musculature. These pathological signs distinguish such cases from the usually observed cases of atonia. Even in the last described instance there were no actual convulsive seizures, if one excludes the temporary appearance of the involuntary distortion of the facial muscles and the prolonged so-called "snout-cramp." Because of the absence of true convulsions in this case, it forms a sort of clinical transition with the usually described group of disorders denoted as atonic melancholia; owing to the great frequency of the latter, and its well known features, I would like to describe below only three cases in less detail.

7. Summary of case history

Peter U. (data supplied by Dr. Kosch, Dr. Skrzeczka, Medical Consultant Dr. Janert and Prof. Dr. Hirsch in Königsberg), 33 years old. Attended the Gymnasium [high school], became a qualified clerk and later a merchant. At home he had already been somewhat subdued and lacking in energy. Contracted syphilis with secondary-stage signs 3 years previously, without residual signs of the disease, but as a result showed increased temporary signs of an already existing hypochondriac fear of syphilis. In summer there were striking signs of a depressive state and despondency, which he attempted, as is usual in these cases, to explain as being related to chance external circumstances, such as business troubles. In autumn he was called to sit on a jury. Became very sleepy, or actually fell asleep during a debate which continued late into the night. He was teased on this account, and developed a fear that he had acted criminally and would be punished for such behavior. After spending 5 weeks in the country with relatives he lapsed into an overt state of melancholia, with fears and restlessness; his facial muscles were flaccid, his gaze fixed. Answered with few words only when addressed, and pointed mainly to his head, to convey his feelings of terror. Evinced absolute distaste toward food; could be persuaded only with difficulty to leave his bed, but even then had virtually to be commanded to perform any movement or action. Exhibited a total lack of initiative. This was followed by a state of complete stupor alternating with a recurrent state of complete disinclination to talk. His talk was sporadic—he would relate how the police had "planted" mirror sections in his room in order to observe him; or he persisted in repeating a single word, in the presence or absence of a specific cause (e.g. on hearing a dog bark on the street he would keep repeating: "Dog, dog, dog, dog . . .").

The patient was admitted to the institute in the middle of November; on admission he presented signs of complete atonia. His facial expression was rigid, the eyes and head always directed downwards; no signs of voluntary activity; remained in a constant sitting posture on the couch. No signs of sensory loss; had to be fed. After various seemingly fruitless attempts to elicit information from him as to personal matters, he gave his age in a soft voice, and even this after a prolonged period of waiting for him to answer and after questioning had proceeded to other subjects. During this process he tended to support his forehead with his right hand, and expressed his displeasure at the entire proceedings with facial grimaces. During slight movements he often broke out in perspiration. His initial poor nutritional state soon improved following artificial feeding. Psychic and somatic condition did not alter in other respects. 1864—at the end of January he began to talk to himself while being fed, at first in an unintelligible whisper. On the following days it was possible to distinguish coherent words from his low-muttered chatter: "stewed steak to eat, stewed steak is something I like"—these words were repeated over and over. He persisted in these monotonous strings of words until August, almost each day for several hours time. His voice was sometimes soft, sometimes almost a shout; at times he would be seated while talking, at others he would walk back and forth in the corridor, or he would walk briskly near a green patch in the garden. The words he spoke were enunciated usually in rapid succession. The subject of his phrases varied somewhat. At first he merely altered the type of stew which preoccupied him; after the stewed steak he spoke continuously of beefsteak, then of roast veal. This was followed by a stage during which he added another sentence to the repetitious phrases concerning various roasts. He tended to add, in the same breath, so to speak: "Song makes life more beautiful," then "Song and love, song and love." Still later: "Song and love, joy is the most beautiful thing in the world"—"Song and love, joy, wonderful, song and love and joy, wonderful." During religious services he behaved most correctly and participated in all details of the ceremony, but he continued to speak softly to himself all the while. In June, during a visit of physicians from his home district at the institute, he failed to utter a single word. When his relatives came to see him in August he spoke to them quite lucidly, even though he had given his usual repetitive "speeches" on the previous day. He was discharged and sent home, where he regained and maintained complete mental health.

8. Summary of case history

Nina von J. (data provided by Dr. Goburrek and District Health Officer Dr. Klokow in Memel), 24 years old. Orphan at an early age; accompanied an elderly aunt on extensive trips through Italy, France and England; returned from her last trip in September 1862 in a manic state. Recovered from this attack within 5 months and proceeded to maintain an independent household with a sister for 2 years. An affair with an officer did not lead to a permanent attachment, but she did not lose her feelings for him, and when this man was killed as a result of a riding accident, she took it very much to heart. November 1864—lapsed into a state of complete melancholia. She spent her days sitting on the sofa, and spoke to her sister only in answer to her questions. Hallucinations seemed to be absent. With respect to moods and interest in various activities, a state of utmost apathy and lack of energy prevailed. Her posture was very flaccid, facial expression subdued, almost sleepy. After some time she refused food. At the same time she still busied herself with some handicraft.

On admission to the institute she showed a distinct pattern of atonia of moderate severity. Sat motionless, head somewhat bowed, staring fixedly into infinity. Did not utter a word, nor reacted to sensory or psychic stimuli. Only when one left her, she would look back in an unobtrusive manner. Refused food. Within one month she only once spoke at length; to a question as to whether she felt any better she answered "I do . . .".; on another occasion she replied: "in Tilsit" to a similar question. In the course of another month she appeared more lively, but her condition again deteriorated, and she had various types of hallucinations. In July, however, she was discharged in a greatly improved state of health.

9. Summary of case history

Wilhelmine R. (data provided by District Health Officer Dr. Maletius). 21 years old. Employed as domestic help with a family. Until this period, she had lived under normal circumstances, both from mental and general physical aspects, but during the time of her employment had to share room with an epileptic girl also employed as domestic help; she left her job without saying anything to her employers, and returned home to her mother in a state of atonic melancholia. She sat motionless on one spot, could not be induced to do any work, and had to be cajoled into eating. Most of the time she spoke little, if at all; only on one occasion, after much questioning, did she answer that the Devil would soon tear her to pieces. She reacted to any attempt to persuade her to do some work by repeating these same words and by abusive language. To all questions put to her by the physician she replied with: "I do not know," and added that she would eventually start to earn her living. In March 1861 she was admitted to the institute; there she presented a picture of atonia of moderate degree, but remained quite unwilling to speak. For 4 months her only psychic response was one of smiling. She then showed rapid improvement, and was discharged at the end of the 5th month in a good state of health.

The above descriptions of clinical case histories should suffice in order to demonstrate that the psychiatric disorder described till now as atonic melancholia cannot be regarded as a separate disease entity; it may be concluded that this phenomenon rather represents a temporary stage or a part of a complex picture of various disease forms. Thus, we have come to recognize that in most cases the disease manifests itself in the first stages with an easily recognizable clinical picture of melancholia; very often the stage of melancholia is preceded by true manic states, which cannot be regarded merely as outbursts of despair, described as "raptus melancholicum", because in addition these patients pass through definite and unmistakable attacks of mania; they present the typical signs of heightened total reaction of the psyche, accompanied by signs of increased self-expression and self-awareness. Although the condition of atonia emerges clinically from other forms of disorders, it may proceed, given enough time, into such a state of passivity or apathy and deterioration of the mental faculties that it can no longer possibly be described as a condition of melancholia: the final stage of this disease can only be termed true dementia (terminal dementia). We see further that in a large number of cases, one of the elements of this complex state of atonia, namely the apparently passive or placid manifestations in the functions of the locomotor system, forms a continuous pattern which has a direct relationship with other cerebral disorders; I refer particularly to the cases described (Nos. 1–5) which exhibited, mainly during the first stages of illness, various types of spasmlike conditions or convulsions, and also to the peculiar manifestations which so often marked the final stage of the disease, consisting in abnormal postures and functional movements of the limbs (cases 3 and 6). At first glance these phenomena may seem entirely unrelated: the epileptiform or choreiform seizures, the tonic, clonic or functional spastic movements, then the more or less fully developed cataleptiform waxen flexibility, contrasted with the involuntary rigidity of the limbs which often offers remarkable resistance to attempts at passive movement (negative voluntary movements), and finally the strange repetitive movement patterns, the aimless "working" movements or partly contracted fixations of the limbs (stereotypes of movement and posture). If one observes, however, how these combinations repeat themselves frequently and how, when they do appear, the combinations occur in a certain sequence which recurs again and again in the different patients, the conclusion must be drawn that all these occurrences have a common etiology and only represent progressive transformations within the same basic process. But even if we decline to establish a set definition for the relatively similar phenomena involving the locomotor apparatus, the regularly and frequently occurring disorders of this type, combined with the patient's involuntary refusal to speak and the pattern of disease symptoms which occur in each case according to its particular course, are all of such import as to form the basis of a commonly recognizable clinical entity with clinically distinguishable features.

In this newly defined group of disorders, similarly to the general paresis of the insane (GPI)—with or without delusions of grandeur—clinical changes in the locomotor apparatus form the main and typical features of the disease; in addition, each disease (GPI and this disease) exhibits manifold patterns of symptoms. In GPI the paralytic components are of many varying grades of severity and type; one or other may be absent in any particular case. The pupils of the eyes, for instance, may be typically greatly contracted, or there may be a difference in their size; in some cases the irises show no change. Sometimes paresis develops first in the lower limbs, in some cases the tongue is involved, etc. Sometimes paresis may be slight and not easily noticeable, while in other patients it is very severe and develops rapidly; at times the paresis appears first after an event not unlike a cerebrovascular accident (apoplectic fit, "ictus apoplecticus")—at other times it develops slowly without such a dramatic, sudden event; more examples could be given. In the same way as in GPI, the spastic signs in the newly described clinical form of the disease are also manifold and varied; they will serve as an aid in singling out clinical forms of the disease as they do in the case of paralytic symptoms present in the group of "paralytic mental illness." These muscular symptoms seem the most suited for naming the new disorder here described. Since it may be concluded that each case displays alterations in muscle tone, or, more correctly, in the innervation of the muscles concerned, I would like to name this disease entity the *tonic-mental disorder* (Spannungs-Irresein), or *vesania katatonica (catatonia)*; this name is not meant to provide information as to the nature of the symptoms and the illness in any definitive manner.

In the following chapters I intend to report on my clinical experience and observations concerning this illness to date; in so doing I will refer to and proceed from the literature published so far on this subject. As to the information from published sources, I wish to add that descriptions of similar cases have been given under various headings, in part under "Melancholia attonica," "Melancholia stupida," "Stupidité," "Mélancolie avec stupeur," "Abulie," and "Speechlessness," and in part under complications—such as "Insanity complicated by muscle spasms and catalepsy"; some cases have been described under the general subject of psychopathology in the relevant chapters dealing with "Speechlessness" and "Voluntary

Function and Muscle Activity." The attitude adopted here was similar to that assumed with general paralysis of the insane; here, as there, although everyone was aware of and recognized the specific disease signs and symptoms, they were not able to classify them within the framework of the psychiatric diseases present; thus, various manifestations were treated as complications of secondary importance.

2
Symptomatology

When we survey the entire symptom complexes of psychic origin designated as catatonia, it is seen (as stated previously) that during its course all the main clinical forms of the various mental conditions may be present, i.e., forms of melancholy, mania, stupor (atonicity), confusion and insanity. The duration of the period during which the different forms are manifested may vary considerably, and repeated transitions between conditions of depression and exaltation are frequently observed. A detailed discussion of this phenomenon would be out of place here. However, it must be acknowledged that not only melancholy but also mania, confusion and insanity may for a certain period form the general symptom of this disease as well as of paralytic manifestations of psychic origin. Thus, these diseases may be classified diagnostically in any of the old groups. It must be recognized that melancholic changes of mood, and in fact all symptoms of mental depression, are frequent among psychiatric patients and that these symptoms are especially prolonged before the transition to the final stage of insanity (terminal dementia). Mania is common in the course of tension-insanity as well as in other forms of mental disease. This is illustrated by the fact that mania is often mentioned in detailed published reports of such cases (e.g., BURROWS, *Commentaries,* 1828; KELP, in *Correspondenzblatt für Psychiatrie,* 1864, p. 322; BAILLARGER, *Annales méd.-psych.,* 1853, p. 262). The second edition of Griesinger's handbook states literally: "The form of melancholy which is combined with mental deficiency may develop independently; however, this may also occur after epileptic fits, following mania, and alternating with these diseases." The symptoms of the various psychiatric conditions are of course quite different, and therefore it is preferable to discuss the time sequence of the various conditions, i.e., the course of the disease, prior to describing the individual symptoms. Somatic diseases whose course reveals a certain alternation, and in this alternation a certain regularity, plus a termination at a well-defined definitive stage, are regarded as cyclic diseases. They are distinguished from other diseases by their more regular and simpler course. Similarly it is possible to distinguish psychiatric diseases with a changing, cyclic course, and others with a more even course. Except for special cases it must be assumed that in somatic diseases of both forms there are two main phases: the phase (or period) of the beginning and development of the disease processes (*stadium crescendi* or *incrementi*), and the phase of decrease and restitution (*stadium descrescendi* or *decrementi*). Depending on the multiplicity of symptoms these main phases are divided into substages: prodromal, evolutionary, etc. It is essential to distinguish the stage of maximal development of the disease process, i.e. the peak stage. These main phases must also be present in mental diseases, at least in those cases where changes in symptomatology can be observed. It is usually quite feasible to enter separate psychopathological processes into this scheme according to the time sequence of their appearance in individual patients. Most mental diseases begin with a change of mood which in itself must be designated as melancholy and which often starts quite insidiously. This is followed by a manic phase; at this time the most extensive mental alteration is observed. Subsequently the symptom complex of confusion appears, and during this phase the signs of mania disappear, all mental functions decrease consecutively, and the process ends in insanity. At the last stage the disease process has come to a standstill, and the symptoms are exclusively those of the original defect of the mental organ. Thus melancholy forms the evolutionary stage, mania the peak stage, confusion the stage of decrease and insanity the defect stage. Whereas the duration of somatic diseases is short, the course taking days or weeks in most cases and the different stages being of very brief duration, the duration of mental diseases is usually much longer, and is measured in months or years. Correspondingly, the different stages of these diseases are of such a long duration that each one clinically appears to form a separate entity. Until recently the clinical forms of these stages were in fact regarded as separate diseases, although it has been known since antiquity that spontaneous transitions occur frequently. In modern times, observation of the interrelationship between forms of mental disease has led to the notion that there are no separate forms of mental disease, but only forms of different stages. These clinical forms in the stages of prognostic course are designated as "primary" or "secondary" when they occur during the increasing and decreasing developmental stages of the disease process, respectively. Melancholy and mania were preferably called "primary" clinical forms, while insanity, confusion and dementia were classified as "secondary" clinical forms. This is not the place for a discussion of the insufficiency of this viewpoint. My aim is to present the fact of the alternating course and the main types of disease as interpreted conventionally.*

The course of catatonia can be properly understood in the context of the above prognostic-clinical scheme. This form of disease in most cases also begins as a change of mood. At first the mood change may appear to be reasonably justified, and thus

---

*A more detailed discussion of this subject can be found in my monograph *Die Gruppirung der psychischen Krankheiten (Classification of Psychiatric Diseases)*, Danzig, 1863.

the disease fails to be recognized by people around the patient. However, this is followed by numerous abnormalities of feelings and of thought processes, or by marked obstinacy, and a transition to other states is noted eventually. It is usually only at this stage that outsiders recognize the presence of a mental disturbance. Thus the initial melancholic change of mood does indeed constitute the evolutionary stage, and this is present in the large majority of cases. In certain patients this initial melancholy is followed by a pronounced maniacal condition of short duration, and only then does the form of disease appear which has received the name of atonic melancholy. It is not yet clear which type is more common: that of initial melancholy followed immediately by atonicity, or the type where these forms are separated by a period of mania. According to my own notes, cases without a trace of mania are less common than cases where the presence of mania, rage, frenzy, excitation or whatever other name has been chosen for this condition was noted at the border between melancholy and atonicity. It is interesting to note that among patients where the peak stage of mania is absent, there are a number who in previous years had undergone an attack of so-called "mania." It seems possible that in very rare instances, especially after very severe physical or mental stress, the disease course starts immediately with symptoms of atonicity. This may occur after a very terrifying experience or, as reported in the literature, after attempted suicide by hanging.

This case is most interesting because of its acute course, the etiological factors, and especially because it demonstrates most clearly the pathogenesis of catatonia. One such case will be reported in full because it offers a very orderly and to a certain degree concentrated picture of the symptomatology of catatonia.*

10. Case history

A 25-year-old sturdy prisoner hanged himself. Almost immediately after the body was taken down, signs of life were noted, and consciousness returned. The patient appeared to be completely quiet and mentally normal. He gave his curriculum vitae and stated that his motive had been aversion to life. The next day he was quiet and spoke little, and on the third day he fell into complete silence. He had a vacant stare, rolling eyes with injected conjunctivae, cramps of the temporal and masticatory muscles and the eyes; he repeatedly raised his hands to his head, and he had a stiff, lifeless, statuelike face. There appeared to be no awareness of his surroundings, only very loud noises caused slight contractions of the facial muscles. He walked about and ate without expressing any feelings or desires. After 3 weeks the patient was transferred to a sanatorium, and some weeks later recovered. His memory was

---

*The case was taken from Spielmann's *Diagnostik* (p. 285), where it was quoted after Meding from *Siebenhaar's Magazin der Staatsarzneikunde*, Vol. 1. A comparable case is reported by König in *Nasse's Zeitschrift für Anthropologie*, 1826. See also Albers, *Memoranda der Psychiatrie*, p. 236.

complete for the period preceding the hanging, up till the moment he lost consciousness, and he described the intense struggle which went on in his mind between making the decision and carrying it out, and his experience during the hanging, when he heard ringing in his ears and saw sparks in front of his eyes. From this moment on, until his recovery in the sanatorium, all memory of his existence had disappeared and he had no knowledge of his return to life after the hanging or of the following period (of several hours duration) during which he had been fully conscious.

This and other comparable cases have until now been classified as dementia, and distinguished from other forms of dementia as primary (Spielmann) and acute (Albers) dementia. But what is gained when cases with diminished or absent mental capability are thrown together on a large symptomatic heap, without allowing for the duration or for etiological factors? How much more transparent this case becomes when we regard—in conformity with catatonia—its rapidly transient symptoms as representing more prolonged, significant states which may be observed in similar cases, and how this clarifies and confirms the pathogenesis of catatonia! We observe, after a trauma which has almost the significance of an exact brain experiment (transient ligation of cervical veins), a short initial stage of quiet and apparently sensible behavior and then a short phase of depression. This is followed by the complete symptom complex of atonicity, initially accompanied with signs of irritation of motor nerves, especially of the upper half of the body. Recovery follows after a number of weeks, with the peculiar symptom of a pause in consciousness for the whole duration of the abnormal condition.

In some cases a short period of atonicity is followed by a recurrence of maniacal excitation or by a period of pronounced melancholy, which in turn may lead to atonicity or to mania and subsequent atonicity. This may be regarded as a relapse of the disease process. Another possibility is that a period of several weeks or months characterized by signs of mania is followed by a transient period of atonicity of several days' duration. In rare cases there is alternation between atonicity and another condition classified as secondary confusion. When cure or death do not end the disease process, the condition of atonicity finally goes over to a condition of such apathic dementia and mental poverty that it has acquired the name of insanity (terminal insanity).

In addition to the cases classified as catatonia which show the above varied course, other cases should be mentioned which develop from a condition of mental irritability or vague general somatic complaints. Here the initial stage of melancholy either is absent or it has hypochondriac overtones without additional symptoms of mental disease. Thus, the following psychiatric disorder appears to begin its clinical course directly with a maniacal stage. Generally the duration of the atonicity is longer than that of all previous phases. This is certainly partly due to the fact that it is impossible to determine the exact moment of transition from atonicity to terminal dementia.

However, although the development and course of the disease appears to be extremely varied, it is not difficult to recognize in all cases a cyclic pattern in the complete course. It is impossible to interpret cases with multiple developmental phases as cases of different diseases which follow upon one another and show smooth transitions. Thus, the cyclic pattern of the course will lead to the recognition of a disease unity, and the multiplicity of the symptomatology must be interpreted as more individual and subordinated modifications of the main pattern. In most instances the disease begins with mild, vague symptoms, followed by an increase in severity characterized by a step-up in the number and intensity of the individual symptoms. The disease process develops up to a certain level, until after a certain period the intensity and number of symptoms show a decrease which persists until the monotony and loss of differentiation of the dementia are reached. Whereas it is obvious that in this cycle with 3 main phases the melancholy forms the first stage of increase and development and the mania represents the peak of the development, the place of the atonicity is open to discussion. In the first place it must be taken into account that in many cases the phase of demented atonicity is followed by a condition of so-called secondary or general confusion, preceding the appearance of total insanity. Secondly, there are cases with conditions of mania which follow more directly upon the initial melancholy and which separate the atonicity from the initial melancholy. In such cases there is no doubt that the atonicity should be classified in the phase of decrease and thus should be regarded as a secondary form. However, the atonicity should also be clearly separated from the dementia with which it was previously united.

When we come to survey the particular mental symptoms, there are few well-established data available on the elements of the initial melancholy. These are easily recognizable as depressive changes of mood, and they are according to observations so far, no different from the initial symptoms of other forms of disease. It must be admitted, that up till now the initial symptoms have not been sufficiently observed, partly because the disease symptoms sometimes originate in completely normal variations of mood and partly because at the beginning there is no suspicion of disease, and hence not enough attention is paid to the individual mental processes. It is rare that specialists have the opportunity of personally observing the first development of mental disturbances. In most cases catatonia is preceded by grief and anxiety, and in general by depressive moods and affects aimed against the patient himself. Very common are anguish related to unhappy love, or self-reproach resulting from secret sexual misdemeanors; this will be further discussed with the etiology. Next in frequency are financial troubles and injured respect (shame), which constitute the makeup of the initial symptoms. It is not rare to observe hypochondria, and moods aimed at the outside world such as annoyance, hypersensitivity, irritation. In addition, all other symptoms of melancholy are often present, e.g. fear of poisoning or persecution, religious delusions.

More specific are the elements which characterize the stage of mania or exaltation.

Surveyed as a whole, the symptoms of this stage form the symptom complex of either agitated melancholy, euphoric excitation, or more fixed insanity. In the first case the signs of melancholy present during the first stage mount to high levels of despair and to general physical agitation. This leads to the appearance of additional disturbances of intelligence (such as delirious disorders of judgment, disturbances of consciousness, delusions, hallucinations), or disturbances of will or actions (various pathological impulses, acts of disturbance or violence). This type of insanity may go along with an increase or decrease in self-confidence, and frequently there are "flights of ideas," recklessness, and cheerful agitation.

The individual elements of the maniacal condition are in part identical to those of the maniacal stage of other disease processes. However, in catatonia some of these elements are especially frequent and of long duration. When many of these symptoms are present during protracted periods in a patient, this may be used as a diagnostic criterion even before the stage of atonicity. The first among these elements is a singularly pathetic behavior. This symptom appears sometimes as histrionic exaltation, sometimes more in the form of a tragic-religious ecstasy; it forms to a certain degree the basis of the expansive mood which permeates all speech, actions and gestures of many catatonics. In paralytics the expansive mood is more often characterized by egoistic pride and presumptions, in the "Vesania typica" by a general sensual cheerfulness, and in other maniacal conditions by a joking mood, a tendency to clownishness, etc. It is doubtful whether these characteristics really distinguish specific types of expansive mood. In many patients this pathetic mood, typical for catatonia, is expressed in the form of constant declamations and recitations accompanied by lively gesticulations. In some cases this leads to the desire to become an actor or to the illusion of being one. Other patients speak about the most trivial matters in a tone which suggests that the subject is of the greatest interest to humanity. Many patients do indeed speak about such higher subjects in a serious tone of voice in the midst of their tendency to perform acts of disturbance, and while leading a life totally lacking order and decency. Often the patients show a preference to speak about lofty matters which are incongruous with their condition and way of life. Many think, without showing signs of obvious megalomania, that society is profoundly interested in the trivial fate of their personality. In Benjamin L. (case 1) a pathetic manner of reading was already noted prior to his admission to an institution. Adolphine M. (case 4) was described as constantly declaiming and highly excitable. Her continuous recitation of poetry, etc. was already noted during the period when the intellectual content of her words was still normal.

11. Case history

Paul M. (data provided by Dr. Botticher in B., with additional descriptions of the subjective condition written by the patient). The son of a primary school teacher, with a hypochondriac and exalted character. He did not finish high school, and became a merchant. At the time of observation he was 24 years old. He had masturbated since the age of 14. 1862 (notes of the patient, aged 20): "After this unclean impulse had been satisfied continuously during 6 years, not discovered by any human soul, and not even suspected by my parents or closest relatives, the catastrophe suddenly occurred." He suffered from hallucinations and delusions (thought he was "Misfortune," "Typhoid," saw the Maid of Orleans standing in her petticoat on an inverted balloon, etc.). He himself says: "I lost control over my mental capacities and for 5 months, while I was fully conscious, the most terrifying things happened to me." He was admitted to the Charité Hospital and after 7 months was discharged, apparently cured. He resumed his business full of energy, but "the germ of the disease had become more deeply implanted, and the secret satisfaction of sexual impulses went on." 1865: "Finally all sexual desires—if not sexual powers—disappeared, after all possible kinds of artificial excitation had been used, while the most sensuous fantasies had been invoked to assist the powers of the imagination." Spontaneous ejaculation occurred. The patient had the feeling that his brain was being torn into a thousand pieces, and because of physical weakness he had to discontinue his work as a merchant. He showed a moral hangover and deep melancholy, and was readmitted to the Charité Hospital, from which he was discharged after 6 months, showing only slight improvement. He did not feel able to return to work, and he could not make up his mind regarding a choice of profession. Because of this "lack of willpower" his relatives requested readmission to the institution. However, despite this "unsuitability for any serious occupation," he wrote during this period an extensive discourse on masturbation in relation to the history of his own life and disease. This was written with much industry after his physician had asked him to note down a summary of the main points. Although the style is very pompous, the content of the essay is quite logical.

At the time of his admission to the hospital in January 1867 he was of rather large and powerful build, in a good state of nutrition, but very pale. During the first few days he attracted attention by his secretive and tragic manner and by his stubborn refusal, which he could not motivate, to go outside the building into the open air. After 5 days striking oddities became apparent in his conversation: "I am in fact a man of fate."—What do you mean?—"Well, things have been hidden from me which were quite interesting . . . my father was a hypochondriac, a closed personality, and my mother was also taciturn."—How does this concern you?—"I have been told that I should become an actor."—When were you told this?—"As a child. I have a good voice."—But a good voice is not enough for one to become an actor; in that case it would be better to be a singer.—"I can be anything . . . sculptor, painter . . . I was quite excited this afternoon; I cried. It may perhaps still be possible to overcome the consequences of the unfortunate impulses and to channel them in another direction." He started to talk about masturbation and after I had stated that he could rely completely on our discretion, he said: "Then I can make my confessions public." This pathetic and confused condition persisted, but the following day a continuously increasing physical agitation led to complete mania with the characteristics of the delirium noted during fever, i.e. agitation as in unconsciousness followed after an interval of several hours by convulsions of the whole body. Fever was absent. During the next 5 days he underwent two attacks of mania daily, each lasting 2–3 hours. The first part of these attacks was accompanied with generalize convulsions, alternating with tetanic stiffness of the whole body and tremors of single extremities and muscles. The patient did not appear to be unconscious during these cramps, but his delirium continued and sometimes he had to be restrained by several persons. This was followed by complete relaxation of muscles, and then by wild, insane behavior with arbitrary striking, shouting and talking. During these states he would often say: "I want to see blood," and he did indeed appear to make the matching gestures such as striking and biting. However, it was always clear that he did not have any real malicious intentions, because he never, for instance, struck anybody near him. Between these attacks he was always conscious and quiet, sometimes slightly somnolent, and always a little confused. Asked whether he felt the approach of an attack, he replied affirmatively; the additional question as to how he felt this was answered by: "I think of eternity."

During the following 3 months mania and apathy with loss of energy alternated irregularly. Cramps no longer occurred during the periods of mania. The mania was most intense, sometimes combined with attacks of rage and an impulse to destroy, and there was frequent declamation accompanied by lively gesticulations. The transition to apathy was rather sudden. Initially this apathy showed all the signs of atonicity: the patient hardly moved or spoke; he sometimes ate nothing during an entire day, and his posture showed marked stiffness and sometimes slight waxen flexibility. Sensibility was also sometimes somewhat decreased. At times he was less apathetic, and such periods became increasingly frequent. On such occasions he would yield some information, e.g., he could not help himself during the attacks— "It is just an impulse, and I cannot explain it at all."—"I lose all willpower." At such times he would now and then employ pathetically exaggerated expressions and formulations, e.g.: "When the principle has been disturbed, one's life is turned upside down."—"I am a part of world history," or he imagined that he was "a great man." A very prominent symptom at this time was a revolting dirtiness (e.g. he consistently relieved himself next to the chamber-pot, and rubbed feces on his head), this being in complete contradiction with his overall behavior during his quiet periods. Sometimes he gave a sleepy impression, not speaking spontaneously or answering questions. At other times he spoke continuously to himself rather loudly. Sometimes he was observed to assume strangely fixed and awkward poses, or he turned around a number of times while his feet remained in the same place.

This was followed abruptly by a period of several days during which he was completely lucid and thoughtful. He started to read again, and took part in physical exercises. After such an exercise in great heat he complained of a headache and developed a condition of somnolence with delirium. When this disappeared he remained quiet, but soon he became more or less confused, and now and then gave mysterious information about himself. This terminated in delusions, e.g., that he was a natural child of his father and the latter's sister, and that this was a great secret. He stressed that these thoughts did not originate in himself, and that if they were not true his mental disease would not be truly justified. He sent his visiting card in an envelope to the aunt in question and expected that if he were right she would understand and answer him. Sometimes he complained of cramps which began in the feet and ascended to the body. At times he wished "to feel maniacal excitation" and he then walked around in his room while he talked to himself in a loud voice. These attacks became more frequent, and the patient spoke vociferously with theatrical gestures, postures and gesticulations. After he had become somewhat quieter but not yet cured, he was discharged from the institution.

Apart from the very interesting symptoms of this case, which will be discussed at another opportunity, a most prominent finding was the singularly exaggerated self-esteem that the patient showed during his whole disease, which was not based on real megalomania. With joyful seriousness he wrote a treatise on masturbation when he was asked to jot down a few notes on his life, and he conceived the idea of publishing his confessions. In the period of attacks of mania and cramps this subjective exaggeration always appeared to reach a peak shortly prior to the onset of the attack: he "thought of eternity" and this was a signal for him of the oncoming attack. When he said that he suffered from complete lack of willpower, he added: "When the principle has been disturbed, one's life is turned upside down." Asked whether he still masturbated, he answered once: "I think that the whole will be solved by the whole." Whereas he had said about himself earlier in an abstract manner that he was Misfortune or Typhoid, he later imagined that "he was in fact a man of fate" or "a great man." He was persecuted by a great secret which he could tell nobody, for it was too terrible. His father was also involved in this secret, and he was a part of world history.

Eventually the great secret turned out to be the idea that he was the son of his father's sister. During periods when he was less mysteriously silent or taciturn, he liked to speak to himself in a theatrical, declamatory manner or to play-act, and this pathetic mood gave him the idea that during his childhood people told him that he should become an actor; however, he could also become a painter or sculptor. All this is very different from the exaggerated feelings in megalomania during general paralysis of the insane, where blissfulness permeates the whole behavior or is based on delusions of grandeur.

12. Case history

Another patient, Julius T., also a young merchant, similarly became ill after precocious and prolonged masturbation. After a preliminary stage characterized by marked melancholy, he developed a kind of religious insanity with partial decrease of consciousness, combined with expansive mania. During this period the patient often became ecstatic and suffered from hallucinations which he sometimes recognized as such. He often showed a tendency to destructive impulses or other maniacal acts. In the institute this condition of vaguely religious insanity with expansive mania persisted for 3 months. During this period his behavior was at first passive and pathetic, later theatrical in word and deed. During one walk he spoke continuously in a pathetic tone and in a low voice repeated the words: "Bless those who bless you"; when asked the meaning of this, he added that if he started with his right foot, everything would work out all right. While seated before a photograph of a landscape he said that he was "studying the secrets of God." Another time—"everything goes well with a man when God is in him"—"God walks in me, he speaks inside me," etc. Once he uttered the following words in a most pathetic tone: "You have certainly seen it, just stand still next to the thing . . . the light of the eyes, the light of the eyes (this was while his pupils were being examined), it must come in the wink of an eye . . . beat on the book (he noted a book lying on the desk). How was the picture—with blond locks—no, not blond—I have seen a picture of the bare tree, and it must remain the trare bee. It is a picture I have seen and next to it I have been." When asked whether he had a headache, he answered: "A soul headache perhaps." During a walk in the garden he held a conversation with himself. Asked with whom he spoke, he replied: "With the artist who made me, with my God." In the case history it was often noted that he held histrionic declamations and assumed theatrical poses. Once a woman who did not know the patient said that an ex-actor had been walking in the garden, from old habit, memorizing his part. Convulsions or other types of cramps did not appear in this case, but the patient had a prominent tendency to strange fixed positions, which appeared during the second stage of the exaltation, and the singular habit of walking with slow, regular, measured steps, combined with other similar striking voluntary movements. At other times he stood stock still and stared at one point, appeared to be in ecstasy and did not speak, or merely moved his lips. He did not develop a real stage, or even a prolonged condition, of atonicity. The state of expansive restlessness slowly changed to a permanent quiet and increased lucidity. During this period there were repeated subjective disturbances of thought processes, but the patient was now able to talk about this in a joking manner. He said, for example, that he still had the tendency to visualize faces of certain persons in the folds of bed sheets; or words formulated themselves in his mind which he did not consciously think up and did not mean, such as "stupid ass"; at one time he felt during several days an involuntary irritation and he was forced to think continuously about irritating events which had taken place in the past. He sometimes had the feeling that his thought processes had come to a halt. Under the influence of mental and physical occupations his calmness and lucidity increased, and after a stay of 13 months in the institute he was discharged as mentally fit.

It is noteworthy that another patient with catatonia fell ill while he was traveling to Berlin to undergo training to be an actor. It seems probable that the disease already existed previously and that the idea to become an actor was an expression of the mental disturbance.

I am of the opinion, as stated above, that the symptom of pathological pathos* has to be regarded as a special type of mood accompanying maniacal exaltation. It is thus a symptom of pathological feeling, characterized by irritability.

Directly related to the above symptoms in the area of affect is a disorder of the intelligence, i.e. the tendency to talk continuously, to read out loud and to declaim (loquaciousness), which is especially prominent in catatonia during the stage of exaltation and which is usually different from the tendency to shout and to entertain people around which is noted in other forms of mania. This has already been exemplified in the symptom of pathetic behavior in the quoted case reports. However, a very prominent symptom, apparently specific for catatonia, is a special type of talkativeness. Whereas loquaciousness in general is also present in other disease forms, the type present in catatonia is characterized by the frequent repetition of single words or phrases in the context of the speech. This is not very conspicuous during the peak stage of the disease, when the repetition might be motivated by the importance which the patient wants to impart to the words in question. The symptom becomes very obvious in the further course of the disease by the repetition of single and often completely senseless words or sounds.

The patient Peter U. (case 7) often repeated single words (e.g. "Dog, dog, dog . . ." when he heard a dog bark in the street) even before his admission to the institute, at a time when the presence of illusions proved clearly that the disease was still at the peak stage. As reported earlier, this was the same patient who during a long period was obsessed by the impulse to repeat the words: "Eating roastbeef is my business" alone or in combination with utterances such as "Singing beautifies life."

The patient Julius G. (case 2) repeated words with a religious content such as God, Love, Hosannah, etc., sometimes in a loud voice, at other times in a whisper. Sometimes single words may change into made-up words or into simple sounds during these repetitions. In Allenberg I observed a case which is quite remarkable in this respect.

---

*[Kahlbaum gives a specific meaning to the word "pathos".]

13. Case history

Matthes Albowski, prisoner from Wartenburg (data from Dr. Richelot, prison physician). He was sentenced to $10\frac{1}{2}$ years imprisonment for 6 thefts and mutiny. During the first 5 years he showed during each year a transient period, of several days' or weeks' duration, of a mental disturbance which could be designated as insanity with prominent religious notions, sentiments and hallucinations. In the intervening periods he was described as an orderly, hard-working and intelligent man. During the spring of the 7th year he again had a transient attack, and in the summer of the same year he developed a permanent mental disturbance of a very dangerous nature which necessitated admission to the provincial mental institution. Here he showed, as he had in prison, a peculiar mixture of partially insane madness and general confusion, of maniacal excitation and apathetic mental immobility. Alternately one of these states would be the prominent abnormality, but usually none of them was exclusively and characteristically present. Taciturnity bordering on atonicity and mental immobility were usually present during a short period only, at most a few days.

This patient was often seen standing in the middle of the corridor, in a stiff posture, with his arms pressed against his legs, staring in front of him, while he talked as it were to the air in a loud voice. Usually only odd words such as "Our Father," "Amen, amen" could be recognized in his jabbering. Often he seemed to give a complete address in a preaching tone, repeatedly interrupted by the above and similar words, and only a few fragments of his speech had a logical content. He would also gesticulate with his arms or make religious ceremonial movements and other signs, or write in the air. At times during this behavior he assumed very strange postures, e.g., with the upper half of the body bent forward at a right angle while the arms were stretched backward. At one time I noted the following words: "The whole of Pogazzer cannot know that my name is King of Prussia, Prince of Prussia, Prince of Prussia, I also don't know, bullet oh no, forever, amen. Nassapingli, nassapingli, forever amen. Father, Son and Holy Ghost, Father, Son and Holy Ghost forever, amen, forever, amen . . . forever amen . . . I give you nothing forever, amen, not in the Church, not in the Church, forever amen, forever, amen," etc.

Nevertheless, this patient was not demented, and only the possibly mor individual innervation of his speech nerves gave this impression of senselessness. He was still in the stage of maniacal irritation, often alternating between atonicity and maniacal agitation. At times, especially when he had physical complaints, his behavior was quiet and he was then able to speak in a lucid and sensible manner about his suffering and needs. Quite comparable to the speech of this patient are the above-quoted notes written by case 3. In this context it is also interesting to note the case of Benno von T., which will be reported in the section dealing with the next symptom. In the literature this symptom is often reported, e.g. in 2 cases classified as catatonia

(KELP, in *Corresp.-Bl.,* 1863, p. 357, and KELP, in *Corresp.-Bl.,* 1864, p. 322): the patient appeared to be in a poor general condition: he spoke High German with pathos but it was impossible to understand what he said . . . p.323: the patient often speaks about a Jewess whom he allegedly shot, and repeats the words: "Shot, knot, pot, knot." Generally among loquacious patients it is already quite obvious that the verbosity is a result of a cramp of the speech nerves or perhaps even of a cerebral center of the speech organs. In the quoted cases and in many others with a marked prominence of this symptom it is almost impossible to doubt the existence of some type of coordinated cramp in the central nervous speech pathways. An additional argument is the frequent presence of convulsions in the same type of disease. It seems advisable to give a separate designation to this typical symptom, which according to my observations is characteristic for catatonia. I propose the term "verbigeration."

Thus, verbigeration is a psychopathological phenomenon during which the patient appears to make a speech which is composed of often repeated, meaningless words and sentences. The words are taken from everyday life and their use is incidental, or they belong to a special area of human interest, often the religious domain. Often the words are made-up, sounding as if from a foreign language, and these are also frequently repeated. The words spoken by the patient appear to have the character of a discourse, i.e. of words spoken to somebody else, with a certain purpose, and born of a certain mood. This is obvious from fragments of the patient's speech, as well as from the energy which he shows in mimics and in his whole behavior. However, the patient is often observed to give the same speech while nobody is there to hear him. When somebody is present the patient does not pay any attention to the impression he makes upon his audience, and he usually does not react to interruptions. In some aspects this symptom may resemble the mechanism of memorizing a lecture. Often during this process there is also frequent repetition of single sentences, phrases, or even single words. An incidental listener to such memorizing might under certain circumstances be unable to perceive an intelligent content and coherence in the words he hears. Verbigeration can easily be distinguished from the nonsense and jabbering of patients with confusion or dementia on the basis of the trivial character of the former, although the speech content of the latter is of course not especially meaningful either. Verbigeration may be distinguished from verbosity because the latter is characterized by its meaningful content and the relation between the spoken words and the mood of the patient. The so-called "flight of ideas" may be compared with verbigeration but is distinguished by the progressive character of the content of the words spoken, apart from additional symptoms shown by the patient at the same time. Confabulation differs from verbigeration in its fantastic productive content. At times verbigeration may go over to one of the above symptoms during the progressive course of the disease process.

The above-mentioned symptom is the more prominent and typical, since in the same disease form and in the same patient a symptom may appear which seems to be its exact opposite, i.e. the well-known and often reported symptom of taciturnity, the main symptom of the stage of atonicity. This taciturnity ("mutacisme" in French) may either be complete and absolute, or relative, partial and intermittent. In its mildest form the patient speaks in very low tones, almost inaudibly, often only moves his lips, or else he speaks just a few words and only in answer to questions asked in a pressing tone. He never speaks voluntarily and leaves most questions unanswered, and he tries to avoid answering by the use of simple gestures. In the worst case there is absolute silence, often persisting for months or even years. The patient cannot be induced to speak under any circumstances, not even when in severe pain. In this context a case of catatonia will be reported where the patient, after a period of intermittent taciturnity of approximately 2 years, developed complete silence which persisted for more than 5 years; only after the use of Galvanic current did he become vocal again.

14. Case history

Benno von T. (treated by Consultant Professor Dr. Frerichs and Dr. Westphal before his admission to the institution in Görlitz), 22 years old. Toward the end of 1862 developed persecution mania which soon became severe apathy. In the institution he initially presented a picture of agitated melancholy with hallucinations and anxiety, as noted in the case history written by Drs. Reimer, Pelmann and Schäfer. These notes show that from the beginning he often repeated the same words, e.g. "Be human . . ." or "Please let me have a few words with my mother," or else both sentences consecutively in frequent repetition, or "Where is my mother!" or "Please let me go away." During the first months he was completely dominated by depressive moods and affects, and he acted negatively despite repeated requests and even put up active resistance. Later he became intermittently amenable to persuasion, and he even started on his own initiative to study, not without success, English and Latin. But by the second month of his stay in the institution he was undergoing transient periods of persistent taciturnity with apathy. There were quite irregular transitions between periods of silent immobility and periods of more or less irritated melancholic agitation. At the beginning of a silent period he did not answer questions but he would repeat monotonous sentences, e.g. "Please let me go away" or "Be human." At most he answered the question as to how he felt with the single word "Sad." Sometimes he expressed something by means of gestures, or he uttered inarticulate sounds. However, he was mostly silent for days at a time, even when visited by his mother or by other persons whom he had previously himself asked to come. Once he was found asleep during such a silent period, and when he was woken by his physician he spoke a few words, but then immediately relapsed into silence. During the silent periods he for a long time persisted in the habit of pursing his lips and pressing them together "convulsively" (Dr. Reimer), or of pressing a hand firmly to his mouth. Sometimes he brought his hand to his mouth only when somebody spoke to him. It often seemed as if he wanted to answer but was prevented from doing so.

During the period of melancholic agitation he was reluctant to be alone. He appeared to be anxious, and showed a cringing politeness toward the physicians and other persons. For example, he persisted in kissing their hands, coats, or even their feet, and only once did he behave in a markedly impolite way. He complained readily and in an exaggerated manner when he had some pain due to minor intercurrent diseases. He often complained of headaches and described them as unbearable. He once told that he had previously often had headaches which caused the sensation of somebody sticking a needle into his head or of a worm boring into his skull. He still had this type of headache, but less frequently than in the past. A few days later he complained of pain in the perineum while he bowed his head forward. He spoke about a secret machine, electrical or otherwise, which caused these complaints. For a long time the influence of this secret machine played an important part in his delusions. He felt this influence most strongly when he was sitting in his room, less when he lay on his bed, and least when he was outside the building. He also said that he felt quite clearly that a leech or worm was gnawing at his brain. Two months later he accused the physician of putting a leech in his brain, or of trephining him with his electrical machine. From the beginning he had the idea of being persecuted, and he connected this with his admission to the institution. He imagined that his mother wanted to steal his possessions and that his physicians were involved in a conspiracy against him. He once showed scars on his legs (of furunculosis), saying that these were the signs of his persecution. He soon developed hallucinations with different contents. He imagined all kinds of foreign admixtures in his food and smelled nauseating stenches, and it was repeatedly suspected that he had auditory hallucinations.

Apart from the alternating periods of silence and agitation, he showed alternating periods of very marked and persistent negative and opposing behavior and periods of complete willingness. During his negative periods, which incidentally lasted much longer than the periods of positive behavior, he refused to take his medicine, to leave his room, to let his foot be measured for a pair of slippers, to write to his mother, to eat, etc., and he listened only to force, whereas at other times he was amenable to everything. On the one hand this willingness bordered on normal behavior, and he was then able to hold a normal conversation and to study English, etc., but on the other hand this condition bordered on apathy and absence of willpower.

From the beginning the repetition of single words and phrases was prominent, and early in the disease a tendency could be observed to assume fixed postures and positions of the extremities. The strangely spasmodic pursing of the lips ("snout cramp") which alternated with pressing of the hands to the mouth has already been mentioned. For a long time he stopped up his ears, at other times he rolled on the ground or sat on the floor, the hands stretched forward defensively. Often his whole body trembled severely and his face wore the most terrible grimaces. This was sometimes combined with complaints of pain. Later he grimaced without any other signs of pain. He often kneeled down outside the building or in front of any person with whom he had nothing to do at all, while closing his ears and mouth with his hands. He showed all kinds of singularities in regard to his clothes and other aspects of his external appearance, and in all these abnormalities a most prominent phenomenon was the persistent repetition. For example, he often kissed the hands of his physicians again and again.

Despite all alternations and the many particulars, the melancholic character could easily be recognized during the first years, i.e. the prominence of depressive moods, and the possibility of explaining his whole behavior from this angle. However, other symptoms kept appearing which did not belong to this syndrome, e.g., unmotivated laughter which became increasingly frequent. Eventually the strange gesticulations and movements, which initially could have been motivated in an intelligent way, acquired an obviously insane character. In the same way the repetition of words, which might have been motivated in the beginning, had to be understood as involuntary behavior later in the course of the disease. The patient obviously showed a transition from the condition of melancholy to a state of confusion with the characteristics of beginning dementia. This transition was probably completed at the end of the second year, from which time he became completely silent. At the beginning of December 1864 it was noted in the case history: "laughs often and without motive, often grimaces, shows many tics, often rolls himself in the bed covers instead of lying under them, frequently lies with his head at the foot of the bed, often retires shyly at the beginning of the physician's round, often smiling, but always silent." Signs of melancholy were no longer noted. However, abnormalities in movements and gesticulation and mimics which had previously been present during short periods only, now became increasingly persistent. In addition his whole behavior had a rigid, negative and tense character (he strongly resisted all passive movements, but apart from this he was apathetic). Acoustically his silence was always complete. However, he began more and more to answer questions and remarks with mimics, later with pantomime, and he eventually used a dictionary, newspapers or books in order to make certain coherent communications by showing words. Again it was quite striking to note the repetition of single words, such as "criminal," "black magic," "noise," "diplomacy," "blasphemy." Once he consecutively showed the words "nurse," "sugar," "medicine," "as," and he nodded happily at the explanation "the nurse gives him sugar as medicine." Finally a trial was made in the last spring (1870) to make him speak by the psychological impact of galvanization. The induction apparatus was shown to him, and it was explained that when the rheophores were placed on him he would receive a sensation of streaming through his body which would also affect the speech nerves and which would enable him to speak again, either immediately or after some time. One forenoon the electrodes were placed on the muscles of the right upper arm and forearm, and current was increased until the muscles contracted strongly and the face showed painful grimaces. The patient bore it with a certain satisfaction, and on the same day he spoke spontaneously to the physician during the afternoon visit. The treatment was continued for some time, and on each occasion he came to the sessions with obvious pleasure and used his regained speech with visible satisfaction. From then on he did not lose his power of speech again, although the symptoms of unmotivated silence, gesticulations during speaking, and the showing of words went on even more frequently than before.

Initially it appeared as if with the speech there also returned some mental content. Apart from the use of fragmentary forms of speech, e.g. the repeatedly employed words "departure for Löbau," he could now speak quite coherently about persons and regions he had known. During these conversations there were prominent impulsive digressions from the subject due to the passive motive of similarity, e.g. "I have been to Geneva, there are mountains near Geneva." Have you also been to Lausanne?—"Yes, also to Ouchy."—"Have you also been to Berlin?" (he asks the physician)—Yes.—"There is Frerichs—Westphalia—Skanzoni in Heidelberg—Graefe—is a famous physician." He was very much interested in names of diplomats and every day he repeated with almost parrotlike monotony the same questions, without taking into account whether or not he received an answer or had already repeatedly received an answer in the past, e.g. "Do you know Prince Gortschakoff?" or "Where is Bismark?" or "Could you tell me something about diplomacy? Could you tell me something about Bismarck? Could you tell me something about Thouvenel?" etc. Once he uttered the following sentences, wholly within the framework of the continuous train of thought: "I have written a letter about Cavour, Count Bismarck became Minister, Prince Gortschakoff became Foreign Secretary of the Emperor of Russia. Have you been to Löbau? Did you hear from Thouvenel? I am a Catholic, the young Archduke in Vienna is also a Catholic." He did not speak very rapidly, but uttered all these words in one breath as it were. He never allowed answers or interruptions and questions to divert him from the flow of the above speech, which was often repeated. Even though the sentences appeared different, the way of speaking and the words were always identical, and there was a striking resemblance to a speaking machine into which certain words and sentences have been spoken, which is always wound up, and which can be galvanized into performing some revolutions by the air movement caused by an approaching person.

When we survey the case it is possible to distinguish an initial developmental stage of melancholy, followed by a period with frequently alternating states of atonicity, slight excitation and agitation, insane confusion and melancholic depression. This went over to a final stage of mental deficiency bordering on terminal dementia, with lingerings of the preceding conditions. No mention is made of cramps during the early stages, but later fixed positions, postures and spasmodic movements are very prominent. Additional noteworthy phenomena were the verbigeration, the negativity, and finally the extremely long duration of the mutism. It was very interesting to note that the patient appeared to be compelled to silence, that he tried, with apparent pleasure, to make himself understood by means of gesticulations and showing of words, and finally that he was most satisfied to be subjected to the painful manipulations which were to restore his powers of speech.

Many patients who have "awoken" from a condition of silent atonicity have said that they did not speak because this was forbidden to them by a voice (an "inner" voice, or a voice which they could clearly hear and which was thus hallucinated). In other cases patients have complained of a complete absence of thought and of a lack of ability to observe. Another group of patients was unable to indicate the reason for their silence. Judging from the first category, it would seem possible to regard the taciturnity as a voluntary symptom, whereas in the other cases it is feasible to assume a kind of paralysis in the speech nerve tract. However, it is also permissible to assume in both cases a spastic condition which secondarily, by means of a reflex in the acoustic tract, causes hallucinations in the same sense organ. From this viewpoint the symptoms of both loquaciousness and taciturnity result from the same alteration in innervation. Loquaciousness and verbigeration could then be compared with clonic cramps and taciturnity with tonic cramps.

The symptoms which have been especially emphasized in the foregoing all belong to the goup of formal disturbances. Another symptom in this group which should be mentioned is the "flight of ideas." In the maniacal stage of catatonia this symptom appears in principle in the same form as in mania in other psychiatric diseases. Another typical symptom is the tendency to use diminutives often and with preference. Apart from other cases which will not be reported here, this symptom was very prominent in the case of Siegmund X., for which ther reader is referred to the chapter on Prognosis. The following is quoted from another patient with catatonia (case 15, Siegmund S.) who initially said that he felt himself to be very small. The quoted words and sentences were often repeated. 21 December 1872: "I have such little smallish hands and feet."—"Doctor, you are so smallish." 5 January 1873: "Oh, I am so smallish, and in two little minutes I shall be deadish."—5 April: "I am so smallish, I am so weakish."—14 April: "Now I am sometimes so biggish." —14 May: "I must dyish, all people deadish, I must cryish."

Finally we must mention here the subjective absence of thought or standstill of thought, which seems to be quite common during the phase of atonicity. This symptom may also be present without markedly developed atonicity, as illustrated by case 12.

Disturbances of the intelligence, especially in regard to content, are less characteristic and therefore less useful for the purpose of distinguishing the disease from other psychiatric disorders than the formal symptoms listed above. In the sphere of the feelings there is a prominence of depressive moods and feelings, and similarly the disturbances of the intelligence are usually colored by depressive hallucinations, images and ideas. Frequently the devil plays a part in visionary or auditory hallucinations and other images belonging to the same group of ideas (abyss, fire, etc.). Often notions of having sinned by having committed certain criminal acts have nothing typical for catatonia; for additional information the reader is referred to manuals containing chapters on atonic melancholy. However, in most handbooks and papers it is erroneously stated that there are exclusively depressive feelings and images in cases of atonic melancholy (or melancholy with stupor; stupid melancholy). Firstly, the cases with a maniacal stage do not only show all the additional signs of mania, such as the "flight of ideas," agitation etc.—quite often there also is a cheerful mood bordering on recklessness, with increased self-importance, delusions with expansive contents, and even traces of megalomania which is regarded to belong rather to general paralysis of the insane. I have quite often noted in catatonics that they imagine themselves not to be the children of their parents but to have a higher lineage (princes, princesses, etc.) and to have been handed over to foster parents at a tender age. I found such notions not only among young persons, whose poetically stimulated fantasies could to a certain degree be held responsible for the birth of such ideas within the range of physiological possibilities (see case 11), but even, for instance, in a secretary of state who became catatonic late in life and who furthermore was possessed by depressive ideas and images. But pathologically cheerful conditions and delirium do not occur only in the maniacal stage; they are also present in the state of atonicity. It is possible to note in such patients that their fixed expression changes into a smile, at times even combined with audible laughter. This may happen after certain events taking place around the patient or again without any visible cause. From information which is later received from such patients it is at times quite evident that they underwent periods with unmotivated cheerful feelings. This symptom of cheerful delirium is also mentioned in the literature. Brosius specifically states that in a few cases of atonic melancholy the facial expression does not continuously show a painful affect. There are patients who even laugh frequently and whose stupor is interrupted by symptoms of elation and mischief. Thus, the term melancholy does not correctly describe even the one stage of atonicity, and it is totally inadequate as a designation of the whole course of the disease throughout its various stages.

Another relatively frequent symptom which must be mentioned is the occurrence of images from the religious sphere, a delusion which is the more notewory since the relationship between religious fancies and sexual overstimulation (which may be observed in other cases too) is very prominent in these patients.

Among the symptoms from the domain of actions and will, the early presence of the tendency to negativism is noteworthy. This may reach a peak during the state of atonicity. In other disease forms the mania is not characterized by very marked disturbances of the will and actions, and there is often a definite lack of will combined with marked variability in both will and actions. In catatonia, however, there is a distinct monotony in the maniacal actions, and whereas the patient shows severe aggressivity and a multitude of actions, this is combined with negative declarations of his will and negative habitual actions. Both in general paralysis of the insane and in the simple form of typical total insanity it is easy to interrupt the actions of the maniac by catering to his urge for change and activity and at most by taking into accout individual peculiarities. A catatonic, however, persists in his own individual manner of overproduction, and he stubbornly resists all attempts to change his activities (e.g. to leave his room, to go for a walk, etc.). In addition to this negativistic attitude as a reaction to external factors, there is a negativism which stems from the patient's own mind and which is typical for this disease. In its most severe form the patient refused to leave his bed and to take food. These symptoms appear to be in typical contradiction to the character of mania in general, but on the other hand they form a characteristic distinction between catatonic mania and mania in other forms of disease. For example, in the patient Adolphine M. (case 4), where the duration of the increasing stage of the disease was approximately one year and where the transition from mania to atonicity showed many alternating phases, the initial part of the manic stage of the disease was already characterized by a tendency to destructive criticism, by a preference to remain in bed and by refusal of food. However, these symptoms are especially severe during the stage following upon the mania, i.e. during the fully developed atonicity as well as during the transition and change from mania to atonicity.

There is practically no case where this symptom of negativism is not present in any form, but its expression may be more active in some patients and more passive in others. A strong resistance against moving is, for example, quite common. The patients remain in bed, not because of some abnormal and pathologically motivated need, but from an aversion to movement or even from a tendency to be perverse. When they have left their bed they refuse to put on their clothes or to have somebody dress them. Out of bed, they remain standing on one spot; they do not want to sit down, and they refuse to leave the place they are in, even if this is a small and hidden corner. Or they refuse to change their room, etc. (case 14—Benno von T.— is especially noteworthy for this special symptomatology). In this form of catatonia the phenomenon of refusing food is most striking. In other mental diseases it is almost always quite easy to demonstrate that this symptom is the result of a motivated decision. The patient may aim to starve himself to death in order to put an end to the misery of his life; he may want to protect himself against poisoning or think that this is the best way to take revenge on his enemies, or again there may be other more or less abnormal motives. In catatonia, however, motives for food refusal are often quite absent, and the symptom is obviously exclusively the result of a refusal to perform any activities which are required of the patient. When a morsel of food is placed in his mouth, the patient starts to chew and to swallow. In many patients of this type one only needs to place the spoon in their hand and perhaps introduce the first few spoonfuls in their mouth for them to begin to eat spontaneously. Other patients eat only when nobody is present to watch them, or—e.g. Julius G. (case 2)—they leave something on the plate from every course; all kinds of similar peculiarities may be present in patients with atonic melancholy. They may persist refusing food until they are starved if the tendency to negativism has not been sufficiently satisfied. These patients show to a certain extent a general negative tension, a tendency to negativism of different degrees, from the mildest one of simple irresoluteness to opposition to all action, and the refusal to eat appears to be only one symptom of this general negative tendency. It is true that at times certain delusive ideas or feelings exist which may act as a motive, as described earlier. But in these less common cases of catatonia with a delirant motive for food refusal one may also ask whether the delirium which appears to act as a motive might not in reality be secondary to the true, i.e. organic impulse, comparable to the scheme of the attempt at an explanation or the reflex hallucination. From this angle the motivating delusion would result from the presence of the organic disturbance which causes the negativism. In cases of catatonia where a motive can be found for the food refusal, this symptom is usually much less persistent than in other disease forms. It disappears in most cases after a few artificial feedings, and subsequently the negative tendency apparently finds sufficient expression in other minor symptoms which have been listed above.

This symptom of the tendency to negativism is related to the presence of particular, more or less bizarre habits in the sphere of movements and body positions and in general in the appearance of habitual actions. Most striking are the grotesque stereotyped movements which may be observed in all large institutions. One patient grasps the tip of his nose every few minutes, another turns his arms horizontally around his head and ends this movement by jerking his hand away. One woman sat down and made arm and hand movements similar to those executed during spinning. Adolf L. (case 6) had the habit of placing the inside edge of one foot on the other and to bend his knees while walking (cases from the East Prussian Provincial Institute in Allenberg). Minna von B. (case 3) had the habit of rolling a piece of cloth in the shape of a sausage—on certain days she sat doing this for hours on end. In the same category belongs the frequent grimacing shown by many patients (case 14). Compare also cases 11 and 12. Another striking habit of the catatonic is his immobile postures, and especially the position of his extremities and other parts of the body during these episodes. A patient in Allenberg sat up in bed for a number of months with bent back and bowed head, following a prolonged period during which she had lain in bed apathetically. Adolf L. (case 6) used to hold his right forearm in front of the middle of his chest while covering his face or part of his face with the right hand and holding his right elbow with his left hand. This position is often assumed when a person wants to rest, or while thinking. In this patient, however, this was such a stereotype habit that deep impressions appeared on the parts of his body which were compressed during this position. The spasmodic pursing of the lips ("snout cramp"), very common in catatonia, also belongs in this category. These typical stereotyped positions and movements are usually noticed only after the transition to the terminal stage of dementia. However, they occur much earlier, and apart from the well-known rigid posture of the patient with completely developed atonicity they are also evident during the maniacal stage, i.e., during the alternation between the manic and atonic states. During these early phases of the disease, or on the other hand in periods of remissions or intervals, when disturbances of thought are absent, these patients are already, or still characterized by the stiff position of the whole body, and by the tendency to habit formation which speaks from their actions and from their whole being. For example, a patient who was in an intermission of complete lucidity had the habit of taking exactly the same route during his walks in the garden, and of turning around abruptly at the end of the path; this pacing up and down was striking for a long period during which there were no traces of intellectual disturbances in the strict sense. When asked why he had adopted this habit, he answered that the sun shone on the other paths, but this was not so disturbing that it would have led a healthy person to prefer the monotony and boredom of this one short garden path. In addition, differences in exposure to the sun resulting from the change of the seasons did not cause any change in his routine.

We shall now deal with somatic symptoms. In the above-mentioned symptoms of disturbances in the fulfillment of desires it already appears feasible to think of a pathological innervation of motor nerves. This assumption becomes even more plausible when we note that certain spasmodic conditions are basic symptoms of this disease. The form of spasm designated as flexibilitas cerea is a very common symptom of the state of atonicity. Other forms of cramps also occur frequently, as shown in the quoted case reports. Adolf K. (case 1) showed choreiform convulsions of the face and extremities. Epileptiform attacks are mentioned in the second case history. Fits of hysteria are reported in the third case, combined with real cramps of the feet, and later of the arms and jaws, this coinciding with the appearance of a sound resembling the ticking of a clock in the mouth. This patient later developed cramps combined with crying or laughing. I myself observed such attacks and spasmodic conditions in case 4, initially consisting of convulsions of all the muscles of the extremities (undulating contractions of different alternating muscle groups) and later of tetanic cramps and trismus. These cramps were also observed in the institution in case 6 and, as in the previous case, there was initially a general tendency to convulsions and later a real epileptiform attack. In Paul M. (case 11) the convulsions occurred over several days, typically accompanying attacks of mania.

Isolated cramps in the upper half of the body were observed in the case of attempted suicide by hanging. In two cases no cramps were mentioned in the medical case history accompanying the patient upon his admission to the institution, and their presence was confirmed only later, after interrogation of relatives. In the literature (as mentioned above) the occurrence of cramps is especially mentioned in cases of atonic melancholy. Since these cramps occur in most cases during the early stages of the disease (only in cases 5, 6 and 11 were they observed for the first time in the later course), it is probable that they are even more frequent than it seems from my observations so far. The cramps were not mentioned by the attendant physicians since they occurred during a period when the patients were not yet regarded as mentally ill, or because the symptoms of cramp were not considered part of the psychiatric disease. Some abnormality in the condition or functioning of the motor organs can be observed in all cases during the further course of the disease. In most instances this is continuously present throughout the disease, in others it is only temporary. In part, these motor disturbances might be regarded as a mental, and even voluntary symptom, comparable to the phenomena which have been discussed earlier under disturbances of the will and of voluntary movements. A part must be considered to be of cerebrospinal origin, such as the condition of waxen flexibility and the crooked positions of the extremities resembling contractures. True paralysis is so rare in catatonia that it cannot be regarded as belonging to the symptom complex of this disease. However, decreased sensibility up to more or less complete anesthesia is common. It is especially mentioned in cases of atonic melancholy that deep needle pricks are borne without any outward signs of pain (I myself have observed such cases). However, this absence of sensitivity to pain is not present in all patients, and in many it appears to result from an inability to react on the grounds of motor disturbances. After the mental disorder has diminished, these patients immediately show a completely normal sensibility, and some retain the memory of the painful needle pricks during the period of atonicity.

A truly common symptom which should be mentioned is a certain type of hyperesthesia, i.e. a usually very severe and continuous pain in the back of the head, a complaint often mentioned by catatonics. In other psychiatric diseases there is often pain in the forehead, temporal region or at the top of the head, but this is practically nonexistent in catatonia, and the characteristic pain in the back of the head is less common in other forms of the disease.

Edema, which may be observed frequently in catatonia, must be regarded as a disturbance of the trophic nervous system. This edema occurs especially in the lower extremities, and quite often in the eyelids as well. Edema of the upper extremities and of the body is much less common.

Among somatic disturbances there is practically always a severe oligemia or chlorosis. Also very frequent are disturbances of excretion. Abnormal conditions of the upper gastrointestinal tract and the stomach sometimes cause—even in the presence of marked cleanliness—fetor ex ore, abnormal sensations of taste and anorexia. However, in these cases it may be difficult to decide to what extent these symptoms may be the result of the mental disturbance and of physical processes resulting from the mental disease (such as fetor ex ore as a result of decreased food intake). The skin often shows increased desquamation of the epidermis and accumulation of epidermal crusts. In advanced stages one may observe formation of hematomas of the ears, but much less frequently than in other psychiatric diseases.

Of special symptomatic and even diagnostic importance is the very frequent occurrence of pulmonary tuberculosis in patients with catatonia. It must be noted that in this respect there is also a certain contrast with paralytic insanity. Whereas in the latter pneumonia does occur frequently, also as a cause of death, tuberculosis is found only rarely, especially in patients who suffered from this disease prior to the development of paralysis. In catatonia tuberculosis occurs frequently in the later course of the disease, but also in the early stages, often in cases where no signs are found of a congenital or acquired tendency to tuberculosis. It is often remarked that tuberculosis is very common among psychiatric patients in general, but in my opinion this is only true for the special disease form of catatonia. It must be assumed that the coincidence of tuberculosis and forms of psychosis, which was often noted in the past, was due to inferior nutritional and nursing conditions both inside and outside mental institutions. Disregarding cases of catatonia, and cases where tuberculosis existed long before the development of the mental disease, I have noted already during my period in the East Prussian Provincial Institute that a remarkably decreased disposition to pulmonary tuberculosis and a very markedly increased resistance to the consequences of this disease when it was present existed among psychiatric patients in comparison with the human disposition to tuberculosis in general. I can certainly state from my private practice that it is only in catatonics that I have observed cases of post-psychopathic tuberculosis. Thus, it seems necessary to modify the rule which implies a general disposition to tuberculosis in all psychoses without distinction, and we must assume that catatonia in itself, i.e. the anatomical characteristics of catatonia and the way of life determined by this disease, causes a certain disposition to tuberculosis.

I have not noted any particular relationship between catatonia and other somatic diseases.

3
Etiology

When we consider the predisposing factor of heredity, it is remarkable that among at least 50 cases which I have observed, a hereditary factor was possibly present in only four. In none of the remaining cases was heredity mentioned to be present, and in more than half of these cases it was even specifically stated to be absent.

Among the cases mentioned in this work, only Nos. 2, 5, and 11 showed a hereditary factor. In case 2 the mother and sister of the patient stated that they had had a transient illness. In case 5 the father of the patient was an alcoholic, and the grandfather committed adultery and subsequently became mentally ill and committed suicide. The presence of hereditary factors in this case is therefore not completely certain. In case 11 the patient's father had a hypochondriac and irritable character, and the father's brother died while suffering from a mental disease. In only two of the cases reported in this work was information on hereditary factors unavailable; in all others it was emphatically denied. Among other patients which have not been reported here, there was only one where the mother had been mentally ill. In most other cases hereditary factors were denied and in a minority no information about this aspect was obtained. Direct and complete heredity, i.e. an evident mental disease in one of the parents, was present in only two cases, from the maternal side in each. Indirect heredity was present in the other two cases; in one of these a brother of the father, and in the other the grandfather, had been mentally ill. However, cases where the parents showed abnormal or markedly peculiar qualities are more common, such as in case 11 and in other patients whom I have observed. It is worthwhile emphasizing these data, since wide acceptance of the alleged great heredity of mental diseases has focused the general public's attention on this aspect.

In comparison it is interesting to note that this negative etiology also exists for general paralysis of the insane, although it is well known that heredity is frequent in other mental disturbances.

However, as regards predisposing factors of sex and age there is a marked contrast between GPI and catatonia. Catatonia occurs at all ages, from puberty (and probably even from the last years of childhood) to the most senior ages; moreover, females are affected as often as males. Thus the possibilities of the development of catatonia are relatively evenly distributed, although there is a preference for early middle age. On the other hand, general paralysis of the insane is known to affect males with a marked preference, indeed almost exclusively; this disease is very rare in young and very old men, and does not occur at all among children.

I do not dispose of personal observations on the influence of nationality, civilization, or of the seasons. However, since these factors are unimportant in atonic melancholy it seems probable that they do not play a part in catatonia either.

Apart from the above-listed predisposing factors, the influence of class differences and occupation should be considered. I must point out that among the cases I have observed there is a predominance of teachers, children of teachers, and theologians. This predilection emerges both in the disease form of catatonia—since persons from these professions account for a relatively large proportion of the patients with this disease—and in comparison with other disease forms since, for example, GPI patients are rarely teachers or theologians, but frequently merchants or lawyers. I shall return to a discussion of this relationship later.

Among the predisposing etiological factors we must distinguish between factors which consist of relations existing outside the affected person, and other factors— designated as decisive—which directly concern the person affected by the disease, without being the direct cause of it (occasional or initiating factors).

Among these decisive factors, two are most prominent, i.e. sexual overstimulation and intellectual exertion. As regards the former, in the male patients whom I have observed, masturbation was very frequently mentioned, usually from childhood, and for a long period preceding the catatonic disease, whereas in most cases it was absent immediately prior to and during the disease. Masturbation is commonly present during the disease in cases of general paralysis of the insane, and for this disease auto-erotic manipulations are regarded to be less important etiologically than other sexual dissipations. In female patients the beginning of catatonia is often closely related to pregnancy, and masturbatory overstimulation seems to be rare.

As regards the second factor, intellectual exertion, I have found that especially overexertion during studying appears to be related to catatonia. Among the cases I collected, teachers and sons of teachers stood out.

The first case which I reported was of a teacher in a village school. After he had initially worked as a saddler's assistant he decided to take up teaching. Thus, during his later years he had to make unusual and thus relatively demanding intellectual efforts. The third case was a woman teacher who was said to be extraordinarily gifted but whose very great intellectual exertion was quite out of proportion to her weak physical constitution. The sixth case was that of the son of the village school teacher, who attended a high school, and the eleventh case that of the son of a primary school teacher.

Since children of teachers are occasionally pushed into a teaching career and are thus subjected to intellectual exertion without regard for their individuality, this relation is probably not without etiological significance. It would be interesting to investigate whether in actors there is a preference for the catatonic form of mental disease, but I do not dispose of sufficient material to answer this question.

With some reservations, very strong religious excitation might be included among the decisive factors. However, this is not more frequent in catatonia than among other forms of mental disease. The action of this factor may be regarded as preparatory as well as directly causative. On the one hand the religious and more or less fanatical activity appears to unfold at the cost of the body unless at the same time a conscious effort is made to preserve physical health. The religious tendency is often connected with a sexual perversity; the latter may result from deterioration of the physical condition, or this relation may be the result of a physiological connection which is not yet understood. On the other hand the vulnerable mental balance in predisposed persons may easily be disturbed completely by a subjective or great objective religious impression.

Religious fanaticism was noted as a predisposing factor in only four of the catatonics whom I have observed. Cases where this phenomenon was followed by the development of another mental disease (partial insanity, dysthymia) were much more numerous. However, I am of the opinion that insufficient attention has been paid to this point in the anamnesis in view of the frequency of cases where religious delusions appear during the disease. The importance of this factor for the development of certain forms of catatonia will become evident from a discussion of the epidemic occurrence of catatonia (see further).

With regard to individual, mental as well as somatic, constitutional dispositions the frequency among my personal observations of a tendency to isolation and contemplation is striking. The personality is usually described as silent and mild, the character as very good-natured and quiet, and the temperament as sanguine. But another mental constitution does not exclude the possibility of catatonia and in many cases the patient is described as predominantly occupied with intellectual matters, as ferocious and proud, or as vehemently choleric. A striking relation between a specific mental classification and catatonia has not yet been found. The relation with certain somatic factors is more evident, inasmuch as so-called nervousness has often been present prior to the beginning of the disease, as noted in the medical history of patients before their admission to an institution. Also, general anemia appears very frequently to form a favorable breeding ground for the development of this disease form.

Among the cases of catatonia which I have observed, there was not one who did not have a certain degree of oligemia. In a few cases a very severe anemia or chlorosis was present.

Secondary or preparative etiological factors, i.e. occurrences or tendencies which might indirectly cause catatonia or which might elicit its appearance in predisposed persons, do not have special or typical characteristics. In many case histories only previously mentioned predisposing factors are mentioned, and among the secondary factors the same are mentioned that also occur in all other mental disease forms.

Among the mental factors of this type different varieties of depressive moods are especially common, such as grief, rage, irritation, injured honor, wounded pride, fear, fright, etc. Among the mixed mental and physical factors such as alcoholism, debauchery, privations, and imprisonment, alcoholism is frequently mentioned, debauchery hardly ever, and severe privations only rarely. However, mental disease following imprisonment seems frequently to take the form of catatonia.

Regarding purely somatic causes it can only be stated that catatonia never seems to develop after acute illnesses but often does occur after childbirth. Trauma and brain disease is only rarely mentioned in the anamnesis of patients with catatonia. However, the radical general changes occurring in the brain after attempted suicide by hanging appear to be more closely related to the development of this disease.

Although the purpose of this work is above all to interpret clinical material, it appears justified, before ending the discussion on etiology, to mention a most interesting phenomen which lies outside the scope of clinical observation. This is a most striking epidemic and endemic occurrence of the disease which we designate as catatonia. I am of the opinion that the mental alterations known as "convulsivity" and the "preaching urge" or "preacher's disease"—as far as these can be regarded at all as diseases—show for the major part the pattern of our catatonia in a very characteristic manner. I hope that it will not be unwelcome that these conditions, which due to lack of clinical support have been surrounded by exaggerated scepticism, doubts, and extraordinary embellishments, will in this way be brought into the realm of sober science.

The term itself "convulsivity," used initially in France, recalls the characteristics of our catatonia, and the "preaching urge" or "preacher's disease," terms originating from Sweden, is nothing but our earlier described symptom of loquaciousness, or even verbigeration.

Regarding the French term convulsivity, I refer the reader to the resumé given by the psychiatrist Calmeil, from whose work I shall quote literally the symptoms characteristic for catatonia.* Preceded by and accompanied with convulsive conditions of different types, involuntary urges to pray, sing, and preach developed

---

*CALMEIL. *De la folie, considérée sous le point de vue* etc., *depuis la renaissance des sciences en Europe jusqu'au dix-neuviéme siecle* etc. Paris, 1852. German translation [from which the author's quotations have been retranslated into English here] in LEUBUSCHER. *Der Wahnsinn in den letzten vier Jahrhunderten (Insanity during the Last Four Centuries)*. Halle, 1848. Compare also W. JESSEN. *On Convulsions among Jansenists in Paris. Zeitschr. f. Psychiatrie,* **VII**, 1850, p. 430 ff.

among the fanatical followers of Jansenism, who, as stated, performed among other things healing of paralysis and cures of deafness. "Many remained during two or even three consecutive days with a stiff, immobile and unfeeling body, the eyes wide open and fixed, and a pale face as of a corpse" (p. 256). "The convulsants of St. Médard started, as the Camisards had done before them, to hold long speeches . . . their mode of expression was somewhat exalted and stirring . . . uneducated, lower-class girls spoke in glowing and lofty terms during their convulsions (p. 255) . . . the individual words often sounded as from a strange language, difficult to understand . . . after a convulsion most did not know what had happened to them (p. 258)." The epidemic started in the spring of 1727 and persisted until 1741. Young chlorotic girls, women, children from the lower classes, and passionate young people were especially susceptible to the mental contagion (p. 264). According to some there were 400, according to others 600—700 convulsants in Paris, and many observers estimated that one third of these, i.e. 150—200, were men (Jessen, p. 431). However, in addition to cases which must be regarded as catatonia, other conditions also prevailed among the convulsants (such as hysteria, chorea, catalepsia, epilepsy). The whole matter has become so blurred by the violent discussions among religious and political parties and by the tendency to mysteriousness and miracles which prevailed at that time, and the episode has been treated so extensively in the literature dealing with the history of religion, that we must forgo a detailed discussion of the subject.

Simpler and probably also more predictable are the characteristics of the preacher's disease, occurring during the present [19th] century in Sweden. I shall quote a few short paragraphs from a sober travel diary, as reported by Dr. Spengler*: "Since 1842 the preaching urge can be noted in many girls, especially in the Smaland province. Along with other abnormal symptoms the girls feel a continuous urge to preach . . . Almost all stated that this unusual condition had started in relation to strong feelings of remorse and repentance, combined with nausea, a heaviness in the head or body, a burning sensation in the chest, etc." (Stage of initial melacholy.) . . . Via a stage of convulsions many developed visions and started to preach. In their mildest form the convulsions consist of forceful pressing of the arms against thorax. In the severe forms there are strong convulsions of the arms and body . . . The face and mimics of these preachers showed typical peculiarities which are only observed in somatic diseases . . . The movements are usually involuntary. The patients state that they cannot help but make these movements. This is the reason that they feel as if they are under the influence of a superior power . . . A more severe form can be observed among "convulsants" who, after a period of convulsions, fall backward without losing consciousness . . . Whereas the convul-

---

*SPENGLER. Ueber die Predigerkrankheit in Schweden (On the Preacher's Disease in Sweden). *Zeitschr. für Psychiatrie*, **VI**, 1849, p. 253 ff.

sions and ensuing sleep are involuntary, the preaching itself appears to be an expression of the free will of these patients. However, if they feel the urge to preach they may be able for some time to suppress this, but eventually they have to submit to it ... The urge to preach may also appear when the patients are completely alone ... This phenomenon has swept through whole provinces in the manner of an epidemic, and groups of people were simultaneously affected.

Who does not recognize in these descriptions the characteristic symptoms of the above-described catatonia during the first two stages of initial melancholy and the peak stage with its typical verbigeration (preaching urge!)? The stage of atonicity is represented by the ecstasy of these persons when they are obsessed by religious fanaticism. In general, histories of so-called religious insanity and of religious fanaticism as a whole show a number of striking analogies with catatonia. However, it seems inadvisable to stray farther from the framework of clinical studies and beyond the bounds of personal observations.

4

Pathological Anatomy

Catatonia is a form of mental disease which often causes the death of the patient, as in the case of general paralysis of the insane. It is therefore feasible to suppose that detection of the anatomical basis will pose no problems in these two diseases. I shall report a few of the numerous postmortems of patients who died of catatonia which I performed in the East Prussian Provincial Institute at Allenberg, of which extensive notes are available. Among the cases reported earlier, case 2 was autopsied in the institute. The findings were as follows:

Postmortem of Case 2

Postmortem 30 hours after death. The head is dolichocephalic and orthognathic. Ears free of hematomas. The skull is very white, and most of the sutures have disappeared. Only the lambdoid and some of the coronary sutures are present. Diploe of normal thickness and containing a normal amount of blood. The dura separates easily from the skull. The cerebral sinuses contain no blood. In the falx cerebri over the ethmoid there is a piece of bone 1 cm in diameter. The arachnoidea is very slightly clouded, and at the left side over the middle part of the brain there is more pronounced cloudiness. Very marked cloudiness at the base of the brain, between the pons and the chiasma. There is no accumulation of fluid over or underneath the arachnoidea. The Pacchionian bodies are minimally developed, and Meyer's epithelial granulations are absent. The pia mater contains approximately the normal amount of blood, is easily separated from the brain surface, tears during this separation, and over the medulla oblongata is colored black. The large blood vessels show no atherosclerosis. The gyri are somewhat narrow, and the sulci form large bends where they confluence. Gray matter pale and narrow. The white matter contains the normal amount of blood, is of normal consistency, and shows no edema. Ventricles not dilated. The wall of all ventricles, including the 4th, is covered with an abundance of slime. The optic thalamus is very pale in cross section, as is also the case with the gray matter of the medulla oblongata and the spinal cord.

Thoracic organs: Heart small, ventricles containing no blood. Fenestration of aortic valves. Pleuritis and tuberculosis of both lungs. Left pleura with fluid and organized exudate, at the right side complete adhesion with the ribs. Parenchyma of left lung containing many nodules. Right lung atelectatic, without nodules or caverns. Edema.

Abdominal organs: Liver normal. Spleen almost twice the normal size, with thickened capsule; consistency not brittle or hard. Both kidneys congested, the left slightly swollen. Adrenals normal. Mesenteric lymph nodes swollen, with caseation. Stomach normal. The intestine is very narrow to the rectum, which is wide. The whole gastrointestinal tract is bluish gray. Ileum with 3 ulcers, one very fresh, the size of a pea, and 2 showing scarring, with raised borders.

The duration of the disease had been two and a half years in this case. I now present a case with a lethal outcome after only six months.

16. Case history

Anna G. (data of Regional Surgeon Feller and Regional Physician Dr. Heinrich in Pobethen, Fischhausen Region), 44 years old, a farmer's wife. The mother of 6 children, she was always in good health and showed no special mental characteristics. After one of her children contracted a very serious illness lasting a week, which caused her much anxiety and during which she did not rest at all, day or night, on 14 April she developed diarrhea which persisted for 8 days. After this had disappeared she became somnolent for a number of days. On 14 May, when she had almost completely recovered, a relative visited her and held forth in a long, religious speech which greatly excited the patient. The same evening she developed an attack of frenzy which lasted 24 hours. From this time on, attacks of rage and frenzy of several days' duration alternated with quiet intervals of the same length. Eventually the patient became demented, took no notice of what was going on around her, and usually appeared to be in a deep half-sleep which was apparently interrupted by dreams.

Etiology: No heredity. Religious excitation during mental depression and physical weakness.

Admitted to the institute on 19 July. Here the patient also exhibited an irregular transition, usually once daily, between maniacal agitation and a condition of comparatively undisturbed awareness. During the periods of agitation she walked about continuously, often sang religious songs, took off her clothes, and showed a refusal of food which was sometimes very persistent, at other times passive and easily overcome, and other similar symptoms. In her quiet periods she was completely or partially silent, her mind blank, and remained either stiff and motionless or performed regular, slow, mechanical movements; the eyes were often wide open and she would turn her head slightly and slowly as if looking for something, her hands spread in front of her with extended fingers. Sometimes she seemed to waken from a dream and was relatively lucid, gave information about herself, and was aware of her abnormal condition: she was sick in the head, her thoughts were whirling; this was caused by vexation on account of her brother-in-law. Sometimes she had the feeling that she had done something wrong but did not know what. In her periods of excitation she was always generally confused. Her mood was never completely cheerful.

Her physical build was rather large, but weak. She was very lean and pale at the time of admission. Pulse was always normal. During the last two months she often suffered from catarrhal diarrhea. However, although this disappeared, she died 14 days later, on 19 November, of cachexia.

Postmortem
Head: Skin easily detachable. Skull very pale and anemic. Strong adhesions between bones and dura, which results in tearing of the blood vessels between skull and dura when the cranium is removed. Dura anemic. Sinuses containing no blood at all. Inner surface of dura smooth and white. Arachnoidea thin and clear, also between pons and chiasma, but very cloudy between cerebellum and medulla oblongata. Pia relatively rich in blood, especially in the smallest vessels, and easily removed from the brain surface. Subarachnoidal tissue without serous infiltration. Brain relatively rich in blood. Cortex of average breadth, with areas of increased vascularity; the three layers are scarcely visible and show smooth transitions. White matter: multiple bleeding points on a pale red patchy background, with a gelatinous transparency. Lateral ventricles not dilated, posterior columns extending very far back. Surfaces of thalami and corpora striata covered with mucus; no ependymal granulations. A small adhesion of the lower surface of the left anterior column. Fourth ventricle also showing extensive mucous covering, and in addition the initial formation of granulations. No abnormal findings in the medulla oblongata or spinal cord.

Thorax: Heart without blood, normal. Both lungs full of round tubercles; adhesions of the right posterior pleura.

Abdomen: Ascites. Thickening of the lower right liver capsule. Gallbladder very large, full of bile. Spleen smaller than normal. Kidneys normal. Uterus normal. Stomach with gray mucus covering the surface. Small intestine dilated in some places, with a thin and anemic wall; in other places the mucosa shows vasodilatation and is covered with mucus; no ulcers. Mesenteric lymph nodes swollen. Colon with slight catarrhal exudate.

This is followed by a case which came to autopsy after a duration of the disease of approximately 10 months.

17. Case history

Julius P. (data of Dr. Grangé and Regional Physician Dr. Pincus in Insterburg; the subsequent course reported by Dr. Ulrich, who is at present assistant physician in Neustadt-Eberswalde), 33 years old. Tax assessor, son of a miller. After he had learned to write he joined the artillery. Upon reaching the rank of quartermaster he became an accountant. Happily married. Physically strong and healthy. Mentally normally developed. At the age of 16 he suffered a mild attack of typhoid, and later during his army service he had a number of attacks of malaria.

Psychological data: In the summer of 1864 P. had frequent headaches, and in the following winter he caught a cold, sweated heavily, lost some weight, and was often somber and silent, because many of his friends immediately upon leaving the army received an appointment in the border police while he had to wait for this. Up till 11 April 1865 he always fulfilled his duties punctually. On this day he became ill with a headache, accompanied with sadness and crying, and complained of feeling as if his mind were hazy; he was very hurried, and ate very fast. Sleep was normal; he had obstipation. He remained silent and withdrawn. When on 11 May notice of his appointment arrived, this was opened in the presence of a witness, with great joy. He was very happy with the appointment, but afterwards did not mention this again. The same happened with a letter from his relatives, along with a present of 50 thaler. On 16 May he was brought, with his family, to his father's house. His complexion was healthy and he was not too thin. He sat quietly and retired within himself, only rarely answered questions, and then very curtly, usually only with a yes or no, but always to the point. His head was bent forward, and he only rarely looked someone in the eye. His head was cool, the pupils were normal, the tongue was clean. When he took no strong laxatives he had no defecation. He urinated only once every 1–2 days, usually when he defecated, and once it was necessary to use a catheter. He always had to be asked to have dinner, and the only thing he took with pleasure was soda water. He slept well; the pulse was quiet and regular, at the most 70/min. His relatives could distinguish good and bad days as regards his behavior. During his good days he ate well, and spoke now and then; on bad days he took only soda water, did not speak or answer, had a slower pulse of 60–63/min, and at night sweated heavily. Later these distinctions disappeared, and his condition became stationary. His voice sounded flat and broken; his muscular strength decreased markedly, but he nevertheless persisted without change in certain postures or positions for hours at a time, resisting attempts to change his position. At times he would remain in bed for days at a time without any movement, while on other occasions he would put on his clothes without being asked to do so.

According to his wife he only defecated after a clysma and urinated only via a catheter. On 19 June he allegedly lost approximately one liter of blood from his rectum, and this caused marked weakness.

Treatment: Bloodletting, leeches, laxatives, quinine. Later, when skin eruptions appeared in the neck, mild and strong laxatives (the latter were completely ineffective, while castor oil had the best effect), quinine and quinoidine, everything to no avail.

P. was *admitted to the institute on 27 June 1865*. He had a strong physical build; his cheeks were slightly red, the remaining facial skin pale with a yellowish tinge. He stood limply, with head bent, in the middle of the room. When asked something, he looked his questioner in the face for a moment, but immediately lowered his gaze, without answering. He let himself be led quietly to the window but then returned to the middle of the room. The pupils were normal, the pulse weak and easily compressible, 128/min. He was incontinent for urine. At night he had to be led to the dining table and be fed, and before going to bed he had to be helped to undress.

28 June: At night P. allegedly gnashed his teeth repeatedly. He refused food and resisted attempts to feed him both passively and actively. During the day he did not speak at all nor answered questions, but at night during an attempt to feed him he said: "Leave me alone, I do not want to eat." He lay in bed almost motionless, only his eyes showing that he was fully aware of what was happening around him. The radial artery was tense and of moderate diameter in the morning, the pulse rhythm rapid and relatively strong, approximately 100/min. At night the pulse was weaker, less short, 96/min. The patient passively and actively resisted a physical examination, especially of the bladder region, which appeared to be markedly swollen. At night he released a relatively large amount of urine.

29 June: P. again lay in bed. In the morning he was again incontinent for urine and feces. At breakfast he allowed himself to be fed. Asked whether he felt pain during swallowing or in the distended region of his bladder, he replied "no" and refused to answer additional questions. At lunch he again rejected food, and at night he said: "I do not want to eat, I am very thirsty" and willingly accepted two cups of coffee. In the morning the pulse was 96, moderately full, at night 84, easily compressible. The forehead was coo, the skin moderately warm. In order to relieve the brain it was decided to use a hair rope at the nape of the neck. The patient quite understood the request that this be done, since he immediately stuck out his tongue when requested to do so, demonstrating his relatively lucid state. The tongue deviated slightly to the left and was covered with some mucus. He put up strong resistance to all attempts to bind his hair together—three nurses had to be brought in to hold him down, and in the end it was necessary to put him in a straightjacket. During this period he did not utter a sound, except for some soft groans at one point.

30 June: Reported to have repeatedly tossed and turned in bed at night and gnashed his teeth. Let himself be fed willingly but did not speak a word. In the afternoon, while in bed, he was incontinent for urine and feces, and this was repeated at night. The pulse was 96 in the morning and at night.

1 July: During the night he tore out his hair ribbon. On this day he ate by himself and finished almost the whole portion. He used the chamber pot twice to urinate, but could not be induced to speak. The pulse was 92 at night, moderately full.

2 July: Defecated several times during the night, while leaving his bed; the feces dirtied the room. In the morning he began to speak as if he thought he were at home: "What happened now, I dirtied myself; send me the maid, dear." The whole day long he chattered away to another patient, telling him about his life, e.g. that he had been a flirt before he joined the army, and making remarks about the ophthalmological patients walking in the corridor: "Look, there goes a blind one again," etc. In front of the physicians he was very taciturn.—Do you have a headache? "Yes." Where? "Here" (indicating his forehead). Do you have pain when you swallow? "No." Do you find it difficult to speak? "Yes." Nothing else could be drawn from him. His voice sounded strangely rough, as if the tonsils were severely swollen. The pulse was 96 at night, moderately full.

3 July: This morning P. was again completely silent. Pulse 90–100. At lunch he ate very little. At night he showed a slight but continuous tremor in both arms, making it impossible to feel and count his pulse exactly. (A similar tremor had been present on the morning of the 28th, but at that time this occurred at intervals of approximately 15 seconds, persisted for a few seconds, and was always combined with a slight pronation of the forearm.) He returned the greeting of a physician entering the room, his voice sounding raw and heavy. When asked whether he found it difficult to speak, he answered: "Yes, the machine which works inside me is so very high." Which machine? "The one in which I am lying." But you are lying in bed and not in a machine. "No, doctor, you must believe me, it is a machine, I feel it working inside me, I feel the pain in my chest."—"I do not always feel the pain, only when the machine is working—you may prove it to yourself." He thereupon removed the bedclothes, bent his legs at the hips and knees, and pushed his shirt up under his arms: "Now, doctor, pay attention, at this moment I do not have the pain—but here it comes." According to the patient, the pain was localized mainly in the chest but also in the lower abdomen, and it increased upon pressure. However, his mimics showed no relevant change. He said he had no pain in his arms or legs, not upon pressure either, nor in his head but only in the neck, due to the hair rope. "Only while the machine works inside me is it impossible for me to speak." "I have to dirty myself when the machine works inside me"—"I cannot get out of my bed only because the machine is working inside me"—"The other patients lie in the same kind of bed, I am sure they also feel it"—"I really do not understand it, but it is the truth"—"I felt the pain in every bed I have slept in"—"The machine is unsuitable for apiculture"—"The worst of it is, my father is a beekeeper"—"I really do not know where I am"—"What will become of my wife and children?"—"Does my father pay everything for me?"—Finally he held the doctor's hands in a vicelike grip and would not let go—"Stay with me, doctor, do not leave me alone." At night he finished almost his whole meal, spoke a few words about his wife and children, and seemed to fall asleep. At midnight he got out of bed, walked around in the room, and talked. He was brought back to bed, but left it again and wanted to go outside. At 0230 hr he was led back to bed, where he bahaved quietly. Another patient heard him groan a few times. At 0300 hr he died.

Postmortem 28 Hours After Death

Externally: Rather marked emaciation of the body, compared to the appearance of the face. Skin pale. No livor mortis in the front. Slight facial hair growth.

Head: Large. Strong adhesions between skull and galea aponeurotica. Skull with sutures and very thick bones, blood content low, dura easily removable.

Dura: Externally pale, sinuses flattened, and filled with a firm elastic (white and fibrillar) clot throughout the sinus and in all branches. Dark red, half-clotted blood is found only in the left transversal sinus and its branches. The inner surface of the dura is normal. Slight increase in the water content.

Arachnoidea with marked diffuse cloudiness, and at several places where the brain sulci confluence there are white condensations the size of a grain of corn. The free part of the arachnoidea between the pons and the chiasma is strongly developed, and below this layer, between it and the brain tissue, there is an abnormal layer which shows numerous perforations. There is slight cloudiness between the cerebellum and the medulla oblongata. There are only traces of epithelial granulations. Pacchionian bodies not very numerous. The subarachnoidal tissue shows no serous swelling. The blood content of the pial vessels is very low. The vascular network over the brain gyri contains blood in only a few places. In most areas there is no blood, and only at the base of the brain does the whole vascular network contain blood. Only one large vein (the middle one) is filled with dark bluish-red blood; all other branches are empty. Over both frontal lobes there is increased adherence between the pia and the brain surface, resulting in tearing of the brain upon removal of the pia; in all other regions the pia is easily removable.

Brain: In numerous areas the surface of the gyri is retracted below the level of the surrounding brain tissue. The gray matter is very pale, both externally and in cross section, and in some places it is decreased in width. The blood content of the gray matter is very low, of the white matter normal. In cross section the white matter glistens due to increased water content, and this is also found upon section of the basal ganglia. Ventricles not dilated, with moderate serous content. The stria cornea is strongly developed, and in its vicinity the ependymal granulations are small but relatively well developed; elsewhere there is no trace of these structures. In many areas of the lower anterior surface of the frontal part of the lateral ventricles there are adhesions, which sometimes form bridges between the opposing surfaces (which makes it possible in some places to place the point of the knife underneath these adhesions). Injection of blood vessels appear to be absent in these areas, with one exception. The velum choroideale appears to be strongly developed, and both glomi choroidei show a large hydatid. Pons, cerebellum and medulla oblongata are normal, apart from saturation with serous fluid. Blood vessels without formation of atheroma.

Thorax: Heart relatively large, rich in fat, myocardium pale, soft, cavities filled with clots. Aortic semilunar valves fenestrated.

Aorta: inner surface very irregular, in one area a deposit of more than 2.5 cm high, approximately 1.8 cm long and 9 mm wide. In three areas the surfaces of these deposits show ulcers the size of a pea, and these are covered with small blood clots. The pericardial cavity contains slightly more than the normal amount of serous fluid. Both lungs are pale, edematous and emphysematous.

Abdomen: The whole peritoneum, the parietal as well as the visceral, apart from the gastric serosa, is covered with purulent-mucoid and in parts firmer dirty yellow masses. The cavity contains approximately one pound of purulent cloudy fluid which is almost odorless. The liver and spleen are covered with a thick exudate, but the size and consistency of these organs are normal. The stomach is very dilated, but apart from this normal, and contains a large amount of yellow fluid and food remains. The small and large intestine, the omentum, and the mesentery are covered with a thick exudate. The lower part of the colon descendens in the area of the rectum shows many injected blood vessels under the layer of exudate. This is also the case with a small part of the intestine adjacent to the ileocolic valve. In the small pelvis the exudate is very extensive, and the peritoneum shows inflammatory injection. Between the rectum and the urinary bladder there is a membranous septum extending from one side to the other, consisting partly of organized exudate. The borders of this septum are adherent to thick nodular inflammatory injected masses. The left psoas muscle is partly necrotic and purulent, in the region where it borders upon the other masses of exudate. The remaining part of the muscle appears to be completely normal. The large blood vessels and the external surface of the vertebral column appear to be superficially normal. The wall of the urinary bladder is markedly thickened (thickness approximately 1.25 cm); the mucosa shows inflammatory injection. The contracted bladder contains a small amount (approximately 45 g) of purulent fluid. The left kidney is swollen and strongly injected, the right kidney normally red, with strongly purulent contents in the renal pelvis.

The following case came to autopsy after a duration of the disease of approximately 2 years.

18. Case history

Friedrich August St. (data of Regional Physician Dr. Weitzenmüller in Braunsberg), theology student, 26 years old, son of a laborer: both parents healthy. Very quiet temperament, extremely home-loving. Because of his diligence and talents, the parson of his village encouraged him to continue his studies. He chose theology and tried to pay his own way at the university by giving private lessons which put a great strain on him. During the vacations this income stopped; he was in great need, and often went hungry.

After studying for 2 years, he suffered an attack of cramps during a lecture in winter semester of 1863–1864. He was brought first to the sick room and later to the city hospital. Here he was treated for a "nervous cramp" and subsequently sent home to his mother (May 1864). She immediately noticed a strange silence and fear. For several weeks he sat, without making any movements and completely apathetic, in a corner of the small room, without ever taking a book or seeking some other occupation. His face was pale, but this alternated at times with a bright, sharply delimited redness. The head was always sunken on the breast; the eyes were only opened for a time and then shyly turned away. He usually did not answer questions. Only after many repetitions, etc. did he sometimes give monosyllabic answers.

Etiology. No heredity. Complete loss of self-confidence and the gloomy feeling of being unable to fulfill his goal in life are the exclusive causes. (The privations which he suffered for a number of years and the consequences for his physical condition probably also contributed.)

Admitted to the institute in Allenberg on 10 September 1864. Not puny, but his state of nutrition was very poor, and there was flaccid atonicity, with a total lack of interest, absence of tension, taciturnity. When somebody spoke to him he fingered his buttons, etc. Often had to be fed, or ate only when the door was shut and nobody was in his room. Resisted changes in localization and position of the body, and showed fixed positions of the arms. Had nasal drip. After healing of a facial erysipelas he transiently developed mania, but then relapsed into apathic atonicity. Subsequently he remained in bed. No signs of an extracerebral disease; showed opisthotonus-like cramps without fever; ate little. Died of cachexia on 2 March 1866.

Postmortem 31 Hours After Death

Body very thin. Livor mortis on the back. Abdomen bluish green.

Head: When the skull is opened, approximately 4 ounces of blood flow out. Skull normal, easily freed of the dura. The longitudinal sinus contains a large whitish elastic clot. Dura normal, except for the frontal region, where there are a few pea-size areas of strong adhesions with the arachnoidea. No increase in the amount of cerebrospinal fluid in the dural space. Arachnoidea very cloudy, epithelial granulations recognizable as fine points. The cloudiness of the arachnoidea is especially marked in a striplike area adjacent to the midline of the convexity and in the areas of adhesions with the dura. In the frontal region the arachnoidea contains a number of thin bone plates, on the left side 2 plates close to one another overlying a large vein, and both plates together approximately three quarters of a square inch in size. On the right side there are 3 plates, each the size of a pea, separated from one another by spaces of the same size. The cloudiness is less on the basal surface of the brain and behind the 4th ventricle, but it is more marked between the pons and the chiasma in the free leaf of the arachnoidea. There is no cloudiness over the cerebellum. The pia shows marked injection of the large blood vessels, but the smaller vessels are almost invisible. The large vessels over the cerebellum also show only slight injection. There is no abnormal adherence to the brain surface anywhere. The brain is in general soft. All layers of the cortical substance are somewhat pale, but there are fine lines caused by the presence of vessels. The white matter shows relatively numerous blood points. Soft consistency, watery shine. Brain ventricles posteriorly wide and long, with markedly developed relief. Slight increase in fluid. Surface of the ventricles with mucoid softened and thickened ependyma; the underlying layers of the brain and the fornix are very soft and almost colliquated. The large vessels of the ventricular surfaces show more than normal injection at both sides. In cross section the basal ganglia are very pale. The cerebellum, medulla oblongata and spinal cord show no recognizable changes.

Thorax: Hydropericardium, heart flaccid. Ventricles with white and red clots, aortic valves with relatively large fenestrations. Both lungs adherent and filled with firm and soft tubercles, on the left side larger foci in the apex, where a cavern of 3.8 cm is found; on the right side a number of small caverns.

Abdomen: Liver normal, but covered with clotted exudate. Spleen not enlarged, also with clots on the capsule. Kidneys pale. Pancreas normal. Colon descendens not longer than normal. Marked injection of blood vessels in various areas of the small and large intestine. In 7 areas of the small intestine, in the region of Peyer's patches, there are numerous small tuberculous ulcers which have in part penetrated the intestinal wall up to the serosa. Cecum and colon descendens with larger infiltrations of the mucosa. Swelling of mesenteric lymph nodes without visible infiltration. The stomach shows injection of the fundus and contains ascarides. The latter are also found in the intestine.

19. Survey of case

Wilhelmine H. (data of Regional Physician Dr. Pianka in Goldapp), 26 years old. This case showed during life the usual course with a stage of melancholy and of mania. An unusual aspect was the appearance of negative expressions of the will (contrariness, negativism in word and deed). The diagnosis was based on an attack of epileptiform convulsions, and on the preference for abnormal, stiff postures, apathetic and immobile lack of reactions, and persistent silence. The duration of the disease was 28 months, and the patient died of tuberculosis of the lungs and intestine. The findings upon autopsy were as follows.

Postmortem 22 Hours After Death

Externally: Pallor, skin tender, edema of lower legs, decubitus.

Head: Skull compact but moderately thick, light, sutures easily visible. Deep impressions of the Pacchionian bodies, but dura easily removable. Dura pale, sinuses completely empty. Small amount of serous fluid underneath the arachnoidea. Arachnoidea relatively strong, but diffusely cloudy. Epithelial granulations very numerous and well developed, but the individual granules are not very large. Subarachnoidal space with a high serous content. Free leaf of the arachnoidea (between the pons and chiasma) slightly cloudy and thickened. Pia mater with a relatively high blood content and a fine, bright red vascular network; it is easily separated from the brain.

Thoracic and abdominal organs: Very severe and extensive tuberculosis (some of the swollen mesenteric lymph nodes are the size of two chicken eggs; the left broad ligament of the uterus shows two cysts the size of a hazelnut; however, no relevant reflex delusions had been observed during life).

20. Survey of case

Gottliebe J. (data of Regional Physician Dr. Hecht in Neidenburg), 40 years old, wife of a small-farmer. As a child she allegedly suffered frequent epileptic cramps, and during recent years she had become an alcoholic. Weak physical constitution. For the last three years severe irritation and mental tension had led to restless dreams to which the patient attributed a special importance and which she related at every opportunity. Eventually these dreams acquired the meaning—which occupied her mind also when she was awake—that she was possessed by the devil, and she now went to confession at least once a week. One night total insanity appeared, during which she was completely confused (although now and then she would talk sensibly), and she walked and danced about the house. Apart from the illusion of being possessed by the devil, other delusions appeared later (she felt as if she were $5\frac{1}{2}$ years old), as well as severe confusion, a tendency to obscene songs and words, unmotivated laughter, destructive tendencies, and at times complete taciturnity.

She was admitted to the institute in August 1864. General confusion prevailed, and excitation with short intervals during which she was apathetically calm. This state persisted until she died of peritonitis on 28 December 1865. Especially prominent was the transient symptom of verbigeration (monotonous repetition of mostly unarticulated sounds), of a change in voice and in her manner of speech (speaking and singing with the teeth pressed together, or humming while she closed her mouth with her hands), and choreiform movements. At times she walked around in a stereotyped manner, moved her hands in a circle before her breast, walked around other persons, turned around on one spot, or turned plates or pieces of meat around, and other similar turning movements.

Postmortem 38 Hours After Death

Body very thin, lower extremities with edematous swelling. Rigor mortis.

Head: Skin very thin. Skull relatively strong. Frontal region narrow. Dura with strong adhesions. Sinus longitudinalis with only a very small amount of fluid blood. Blood content normal. Inner surface on the left side shows a thin skinlike covering, in some areas with small amounts of patchily distributed exudate. The same exudate is present over the basal parts of the frontal lobes and over the lateral and upper parts of the parietal lobes. Occipital lobes free of this.

Arachnoidea without epithelial granulations; slight diffuse cloudiness. Over the base of the brain there is cloudiness only in the area of the Sylvian fossa, where it is relatively severe (more so than over the convexity); the free leaf between the pons and chiasma shows a few foci of cloudiness and thickening, and this leaf is very small. The free leaf behind the 4th ventricle is not thickened or clouded. No increased amount of fluid in the subarachnoid space. The pia has a normal blood content (perhaps slightly less); adherence to the brain is normal everywhere.

Brain: Gyri relatively numerous. Gray matter of a strange yellowish gray hue. There appears to be a decreased blood content. The different layers cannot be recognized. Width slightly decreased. No blood vessels distinguishable. The white matter shows relatively abundant, but small, blood points in cross section. It has a strange sheen, something between that of fat and of water. The consistency is normal and regular. The surfaces of the ventricles show no granulations, but the ependyma in the area of the posterior part of the striae corneae is strangely white and cloudy, so that it stands out very clearly from the underlying gray matter. Water content of ventricles not increased. The posterior columns are similar on both sides, of average length. Plexus normal. The gray matter of the large ganglia and cortex is slightly grayish yellow and pale. Cerebellum, pons and medulla normal. The substantia nigra is small and stains very dark.

Thorax: Hydropericardium. Heart small, muscle very darkly stained. Left ventricle with a relative abundance of white clots. No fibrin. For the rest, lungs normal, slightly adherent on both sides; pleural cavities with a serous exudate.

Over the middle part of the left lung there is an area of hydropically swollen connective tissue, extending like a transverse belt over the external surface. Lung tissue normal.

Abdomen: Abdominal cavity not depressed, filled with a large amount of cloudy milky fluid. Liver of normal size, its tissue dark. The surface is adherent to the diaphragm. The spleen, slightly smaller than normal, is also adherent to the surrounding parts of the peritoneum; the capsule is very thick. The splenic tissue appears to be normal. The intestine is not distended, and quite regular in size and strength. The small intestine is relatively pale, and the loops stick together, without recognizable traces of inflammation. The intestine contains a few ascarides; on only one area does the mucosa show marked injection and an ulcer which has not yet healed. In a number of other regions, apparently corresponding to Peyer's patches, there is loss of substance without changes in the surrounding tissues (there is thinning of the mucosa in patches 1.8–2.5 cm long and 0.6–0.9 cm wide). The colon is externally faintly gray, and over its whole length the mucosa has a pale gray color.

Genital organs: Severe depression of the uterus, with prolapse of the vagina. Uterus slightly enlarged and pale. Both salpinges have been displaced from their normal position so that they are in contact over the middle part of the posterior margin of the uterus; they are adherent to the uterus in this area, and there is a cyst the size of a hazelnut, bluish in color, which contains a soft, yellow, pasty mass which protrudes when pressure is exerted on the cyst. In another place a glassy white mucoid substance is expressed. The ovaries lie right next to the uterus. Neither the fimbriae nor the external openings of the salpinges can be found.

Kidneys: Both, especially the right, smaller than normal, with an irregular granular surface. The capsule cannot be easily removed. The cross section is hyperemic, irregular with a narrow cortex. Pyramids not streaked.

Stomach: Inner surface swollen covered with mucus.

Finally I shall report the postmortem of a case where death occurred after a 7-year duration of the disease. During life the patient had undergone repeated periods of maniacal excitation in the developmental stage of the disease; highly developed flexibilitas cerea and verbigeration were characteristic for the period of atonicity, which lasted a number of years.

21. Postmortem

Head: Dura markedly folded in its anterior part (atrophy of the brain), arachnoidea slightly cloudy over the convexity (cloudiness is more severe in only one area, around the Pacchionian bodies). Over the point of the lower pole of the brain the dura and arachnoidea are adherent due to a mucoid felty mass. The free leaf of the arachnoidea between the pons and chiasma is thickened. The blood content of the pia is normal, and there is no external hydrocephalus. Brain small, firmer than normal, poor in blood. The whole inner surface shows small glistening granulations the size of corn grains. Small amount of serum.

Thorax: Lungs adherent on both sides, with tuberculous caverns. Heart very small. Aorta with beginning atheromatous degeneration.

Abdomen: Liver, spleen and kidneys normal. No ascites. Slight edema of the feet.

The body is very thin.

When summarizing the main findings of the above reported autopsies, it is advisable to take into account the differences in duration of the disease until death. There is a series of cases which show a duration of 6, 16, 26 and 28 months, and $4\frac{1}{2}$, 6 and 7 years, i.e.:

I:	6 months	in case 16 (Anna G.)
II:	16 months	in case 17 (Julius P.)
III:	26 months	in case 18 (Friedrich St.)
IV:	28 months	in case 19 (Wilhelmine H.)
V:	$4\frac{1}{2}$ years	in case 20 (Gottliebe J.)
VI:	6 years	in case 2 (Julius G.)
VII:	7 years	in case 21.

Starting with the main organ, the brain, with its inner parts, we see that in two cases of short duration (I, III) and in one of longer duration (VI) the inner surface of the brain ventricles has an extensive mucoid exudate, whereas among the three next younger cases (II, IV, V) this proliferation of the ependymal substance is extensive only in the area of the striae corneae. In addition, the two youngest cases already show the beginning development of the well-known ependymal granulations (in the 4th ventricle in I, in the vicinity of the striae corneae in II), and in the oldest case (VII) the whole surface of the brain ventricles is covered with small glistening granulations. In addition, localized adhesions of the lateral wall of the anterior columns were noticed in the two youngest cases, highly developed in case 2, where the vascular layer (velum choroideale) was more than normally developed, whereas in the third case the high blood content of the blood vessels coursing through the ventricles was prominent. In no case was there important dilatation of the ventricles, and only one case (IV) showed a slight general dilatation. In two younger cases (I, III) the posterior columns extended far posteriorly, a finding which is known to be due to individual variations.

It is not difficult to combine these findings and to regard them as partial phenomena of a process. Virchow* regarded the granulations as thickenings of the ependyma due to a fibrinous exudate in the ependymal tissue. "They consist of the same connective tissue substance as the ependyma itself, but they are firmer, more solid, and tougher." The reported findings represent a continuous series of this process. In the younger cases we see the massive, soft mucoid exudate, in the oldest cases the organization of this exudate to firm, formed structures. Depending whether this process progresses more or less rapidly and vigorously, young cases may show the beginning of the late stages (or less frequently only the local beginning of this process). As Virchow noted, these formations occur without increase in the amount of watery fluid in the ventricles. On the contrary, they appear to offer a certain resistance to the outward pulling forces which accompany the later atrophy of the brain tissue and which cause dilatation of the ventricles. This resistance suffices to prevent the dilatation with an increase in the amount of fluid which is so often observed in other forms of mental disease.

The brain is in most cases of normal consistency. In only one case (III) increased softness, especially of the central structures, was noted, and in a case characterized by a long duration of the disease (VII) the resistance of the whole brain was increased (at the age of 36 years). In cross section the white matter is in the younger cases typically glistening and transparent corresponding to saturation with water. This was not noticed in the two oldest cases (VI and VII). The blood content of the brain is slightly increased in the two youngest cases (I and III), in the oldest case (VII) markedly decreased, whereas in the remaining cases it appears normal or only slightly abnormal. As regards the size of the brain, this was noted to be smaller in the oldest cases, while no change was observed in most of the younger cases. In the case (VI) showing the longest duration except for one other, the gyri and the cross section of the cortical substance are narrow and the sulci form large bends at the points where they meet; in another, younger, case (II) the surface of numerous gyri lies below the level of that of the surrounding brain tissue.

These findings regarding changes in the brain demonstrate the stages of a continuous process. In the younger cases we see signs of a certain hyperplasia, slight swelling, high blood content and saturation of the tissue, in the cases of average duration a more normal condition as regards the listed findings (transition phase), and in the older cases a general decrease in size of the brain tissue and a reduction of blood content. In some younger cases the final outcome of this process is already indicated in limited areas.

Let us now regard the outer surface of the brain and the cerebral membranes. The vascular membrane of the brain, the pia, shows in most of the young cases a relatively high blood content; in particular the network of small vessels is very

---

*VIRCHOW. Ueber das granulirte Aussehen der Gehirnventrikel (On the Granular Aspect of the Brain Ventricles). *Zeitschr. f. Psychiatrie,* **III,** 242, 1846.

dense and clearly injected. In the oldest cases the blood content is low or not abnormal. In only one of the younger cases (II), which in other aspects is also characterized by the more rapid progression of the process, is the vascular membrane poor in blood, especially over the convexity, whereas the pia shows a normal blood content over the base of the brain. In addition, this membrane can be easily removed in all younger cases; an adhesion was found over the surface of the temporal lobe only in the second case. With regard to the arachnoidea, in only one of the young cases (III) was a marked cloudiness seen over the convexity, in a bandlike area adjacent to the midline, whereas in the other cases the convexity is either completely clear and limpid (I) or shows only very diffuse slight cloudiness or single, grain-sized areas of increased cloudiness. On the other hand, all cases show a more or less extensive cloudiness over the base, and especially the free leaf of the arachnoidea, extending from the pons to the chiasma and to the frontal lobes of the brain, is the site of this intramembranous accumulation of exudate. In one case (V) where cloudiness was only slight at this site, a more pronounced cloudiness was found over the Sylvian fossa, and there was also only slight diffuse cloudiness over the convex upper surface. In the youngest case (disease of almost 6 months' duration) the arachnoidea was also free of cloudiness at the base of the cerebrum, and only the free leaf behind the 4th ventricle underneath the cerebellum was markedly cloudy, whereas all the other cases above showed no or only very slight cloudiness at this site. The importance of this finding of the localization and intensity of the cloudiness of the arachnoidea becomes evident only when we compare this with the findings in other forms of disease, where the anatomical relations have been studied in this context. We shall report the findings in a few cases, with special emphasis on the arachnoidea.

22. Case history

Ferdinand Suttkus, 42 years old, railroad employee, was dismissed from his post on 1 July 1864 because of poor hearing. After a phase with symptoms of melancholy he developed typical general paralysis with megalomania, and he died after a little more than 6 months.

Postmortem: The skull is firmly attached to the dura by the Pacchionian bodies. External surface of dura rich in blood; in the region of the base of the right occipital pole there is a thin layer of extravasation between the dura and the skull. The dura itself is of a dirty shade. Inside there is over the whole lower half of the right side of the cerebrum a pachymeningitic extravasation which is partly very thin and partly slightly thicker. The sinuses contain a small amount of clotted blood. No external hydrocephalus. Arachnoidea very cloudy, especially over the upper and lower parts of the right hemisphere, and also over all parts of the base where a subarachnoidal space is present; the free leaf is only slightly cloudy. Meyer's epithelial granulations are extended over the whole brain surface. Pacchionian bodies relatively strongly developed, but only on the borders of the median cleft. Pia moderately rich in blood, easily removable. External size of the brain not decreased. Gray matter with distinct layers, mostly pale; in some areas the inner layer shows marked injection. White matter with average blood content. Ventricles dilated, with abundant fluid. The whole surface is covered with ependymal granulations. Stria cornea strongly developed. Fourth ventricle rich in granulations; in the vicinity of the floor dark blue injection of vessels is marked. Large ganglia of normal color and consistency. Cerebellum with swollen gray gelatinous and transparent cortex and narrowed white matter. No changes in the vessels of the brain or of the plexus.

Spinal cord: Dura markedly hyperemic; externally from the dura in the middle part of the back there is a hemorrhagic membranous exudate. Arachnoidea with gelatinous infiltration in the posterior half, strongly adherent to the dura. Underneath the arachnoidea a gray band shines through on each side over the whole length. Cross section of the spinal cord of normal size; the gray matter of the posterior columns appears widened, especially at the periphery. This gray matter is soft and transparent. Its degeneration is especially marked in the lower third.

If we disregard all other findings, we see after a disease of only slightly more than 6 months' duration already marked cloudiness of the whole arachnoidea, especially in the anterior parts of the convexity and over the base, less in the leaf between the pons and chiasma, and elsewhere in isolated areas. This is combined with epithelial granulations and important changes in the dura mater. Another case is cited below.

23. Case history

Reinhold Schukat, 44 years old, laborer. In the middle of January 1864 he has to join a large hunting party as a servant. He is healthy when he leaves, but on his return 7 days later he is taciturn, and when he begins to speak again he shows megalomania and paralysis. This is soon followed by rage and a rapid decrease in intelligence. Dies on 25 January of the following year, the disease having lasted for something less than one year.

Autopsy: Skull normally developed, poor in blood. Dura externally normal. Sinuses containing a few clots. When the subdural space is opened, a great deal of fluid flows out, and afterward the membrane lies folded on the brain. Upon removal of the dura from the convexity a mucoid-fibrillar membrane is noted which is connected to the dura in some areas, detaches from the dura, and remains lying on the arachnoidea. This membrane is not continuous and appears to have no blood vessels. On the inner surface of the dura over the right frontal and parietal areas fresh flat extravasations are noted, mostly in the right frontal area, where they appear to be oldest. Both posterior fossae show a small amount of rust-colored exudate. Arachnoidea over the whole convexity strongly cloudy, regular and diffuse; in three areas there is a caseous-white thickening the size of a pea. Epithelial granulations only weakly developed, but present all over the convexity. At the base the arachnoidea is very cloudy over the Sylvian fossa, less so over the angle between the pons and chiasma, regular and without thickening. Over the 4th ventricle there is also slight cloudiness. The subarachnoidal tissue shows a strong serous infiltrate. The pia appears to be more adherent than usual to the brain, since brain tissue is torn off when this membrane is removed. Eventually it is possible to remove the membrane everywhere. The pial blood vessels are mostly injected and form a dense network, but in one area in the right half of the skull the vessels are completely empty. Larger vessels moderately filled; in the basilar artery a partly white, soft clot; no visible atheromas, but the vascular walls appear to be very tough. Gyri numerous but narrow. Sulci not widened, lying between the gyri as is normal. Brain substance slightly firmer than normal (this probably caused the increased adhesion due to the connecting vessels which were revealed when the pia was removed). Gray matter dark, in many areas very narrow; in many places the inner layer is very red. In cross section the centrum semiovale shows an average blood content and glistens brightly. Ventricles not dilated. Posterior columns shorter than usual. The surface of the ventricles has a thickened ependyma and ependymal granulations. Cerebellum, medulla oblongata and spinal cord (as far as the latter can be reached from the cranial cavity) without abnormalities. Plexus without cysts.

Here we again find—except for the extensive pachymeningitis—after only one year marked cloudiness of the arachnoidea, especially on the convexity; similar strong cloudiness at the base is present only over the Sylvian fossa, whereas the free leaf is much less affected.

Two more cases of general progressive paralysis with megalomania will be mentioned briefly.

24. Summary of case

Julius N., 31 years old, an assessor, fell ill at the end of 1863. He showed the most common symptoms of paralytic mental disturbance, with rapid development of signs of paralysis, and he died in September 1865.

Autopsy: The dura shows many remaining traces of pachymeningitis over the whole right convexity, and also on the left side and over the base of the brain. Over the convexity the entire arachnoidea is very cloudy, which gives a tendonlike white appearance to the whole membrane. On the base there are only a few small patches, and there are larger bands along the vessels. Over the convexity the thickness and strength of the arachnoidea are markedly increased. The free leaf in front of the pons and the free leaf behind the 4th ventricle are only slightly thickened. Pacchionian bodies strongly developed along the median cleft, the epithelial granulations only slightly developed. Ependymal granulations only present in the 4th ventricle.

25. Case history

Julius von O., 35 years old, a railroad official, became ill after an epileptic attack in June 1862 and a repetition in May 1863. The disease started after the latter attack, and the patient showed difficulties in moving the tongue, deafness, and progressive paralysis with a very prominent decrease in intelligence. After hospitalization for 6 months in an institution he had a remission which enabled him to return to his job for half a year. Recurrent epileptic attacks then led to profound dementia and finally, in November 1865, to his death.

Autopsy: Pachymeningitis with only slightly developed membranes at the base and over the frontal lobes. Over the convexity the whole arachnoidea is transformed into a regular paperlike membrane. At the base this change has occurred only over the larger sulci and over the angle between the pons and chiasma. Epithelial granulations small but present everywhere. Pacchionian bodies small but very numerous along the median cleft. Subarachnoidal tissues greatly swollen. Ventricles dilated, hydropic. Ependyma thickened only at the stria. Ependymal granulations numerous but small.

Whereas in both of the younger cases with a duration of the disease of less than one year the cloudiness of the arachnoidea has already progressed to the same degree as in the oldest cases of catatonia, the arachnoidea in the older cases (duration 2 and $2\frac{1}{2}$ years) is white and resembles a tendon, i.e. not only cloudy but opaque, condensed to resemble paper, and firm. In addition this cloudiness is very extensive, encompassing the whole convexity (if it spreads to the base, its intensity and extent are much less). In catatonia, however, there is in some cases cloudiness only at the base, and in only one case (III) was there marked participation of the convexity in the form of circumscribed streaks.

In accordance with the lesser deposition of exudate in the arachnoideal membrane, the development of Meyer's epithelial granulations is also only very slight in catatonia. Only one case (III) revealed formation of bone plates, in an area where the dura was adherent to the arachnoidea, so that it is probable that this bone formation was derived from the dura, which is very often the site of such changes. In another case (V) we also find bone formation in the falx cerebri immediately over the ethmoid crista. It may be of importance that in both these cases in which bone plates were present in the meningeal membranes, the first signs of disease during life had been epileptic convulsions.

Apart from the above-mentioned changes, the dura showed another abnormality in one case, i.e. a thin skinlike exudate on the inner surface (case V, after a duration of the disease of approximately 4 ½ years). If we compare this with the findings in the other four cases reported, who all showed traces of extensive pachymeningitis which must have occurred early in the disease and must have rapidly developed in intensity, this also has to be recognized as an important difference between GPI and catatonia.

The blood content of the skull was decreased in some cases of catatonia, but normal in others. In the second case, interesting because of the intensity of its development, the thickness of the skull was prominent in this young individual; in another case (IV) the sutures had disappeared.

With regard to the extracranial organs it is noteworthy that except for one case with emphysema of the lungs (II), all cases had tuberculosis of the lungs and the abdominal organs, usually very extensive.

If we now review all the data derived from the anatomical findings, we see that in almost all tissue components of the intracranial organs—at least of those where important changes were at all regularly found—a genetically coherent process was observed. The developmental stages of this process were able to be followed in the cases of different duration. In younger cases we found more marked congestion of blood in the free vessels of both the outer and the inner surface of the brain, combined with serous saturation and softening of the tissue without a decrease in the size of the brain, but with formation of exudate on the inner surface and in the outer lining, the arachnoidea, with a preference for deposition at the base. In the older cases the blood congestion disappeared, but there was a decrease in size (retraction) of the brain and organization of the whole soft ependymal exudate to dry granulations. In the surrounding cerebral membranes which, especially in older cases, are usually the site of major processes, we find only very slight changes. The results of pachymeningitis exudation in the form of more or less developed rust-colored membranes on the inside of the dura, which are so common in the most diverse forms of mental disease, and the thick tumorous hematomas that are very frequent in general paralysis of the insane with or without megalomania, are rare in catatonia, according to my observations. Among the reported postmortems there is only one case (V) showing a mild degree of a comparable change, despite the duration of the disease.

The arachnoidea is more regularly the site of changes. Only in the youngest case was the cloudiness of this membrane limited to the free leaf between the cerebellum and medulla oblongata (behind the 4th ventricle). In all the other cases at least the free leaf of the arachnoidea between the pons and chiasma was more or less cloudy, and in some cases this area was exclusively or most severely affected in the form of single streaks. In some cases there are two superimposed leaves at this site. We have already drawn attention to the noteworthy tendency of this exudate to be deposited in the direction of the base. This predilection for cloudiness of the basal arachnoidea is also in accordance with the weak development of the Pacchionian bodies in catatonia, whereas these (as well as cloudiness of the convexity) are very markedly developed in other mental diseases.

If we attempt to classify the above findings according to their significance, we have to isolate the phenomena which refer to mental disturbances in general from those elements which are specific to this special form of disease. Most if not all mental diseases of cerebral origin result from disturbances of nutritional processes; in most cases these show initially signs of intensification (hyperemia, swelling, exudation), and after a longer duration and at the end of the process signs of regression and diminution (atrophy, hydrops, formation of neoplasms). The bulk of the anatomical findings in the body of a patient who has died while suffering from a mental disease refer to such processes, which are to a certain extent general. The number of changes noted in each case is known to be as a rule relatively high in cases where the disease has not rapidly led to death. Many of the symptoms in a large number of cases of prolonged mental disease are probably based on these general processes. In particular, cases which during the first stage showed more or less marked states of irritation and increased function, to be followed by a tendency to general mental deterioration (terminal dementia), can probably be correlated with these degenerative nutritional processes. In this context the individual anatomical changes are probably not important, just as for the clinical observation of the disease the special mental characteristics or the pathological content of the delusions of each case are only of minor significance.

In addition to these general processes—and also within these processes—we must isolate those elements and factors which, according to experience and statistical studies, have a closer relation to special forms of disease or disease courses or to individual symptomatic mental conditions. For catatonia, which is also based on the general process of degeneration leading through initial hyperplasia to eventual atrophy, the highly transient nature and slight intensity of the signs of congestion in the first phase must be regarded as characteristic. The second phase shows a late occurrence of the retraction (atrophy) of the brain tissue, related to the absence of significant dilatation of the ventricles. In progressive general paralysis, the only organic psychosis which can be used as an object of comparison in view of the present development of pathological anatomy, the first stage of the general degenerative process is characterized by very prominent hyperemia and massive exudates, whereas the atrophy develops soon afterward. In an early stage the cortical substance shows defects, and in addition the white substance also retracts, resulting in the formation of cavities. A further typical difference in catatonia is found in the limited extent and in the direction of deposition of exudates in the cerebral membranes, especially in the arachnoidea where, as stated above, the base shows relatively dense and more frequent cloudiness and where the free leaf extending from the pons to the chiasma and the frontal lobes, and the area lying in a band adjacent to the Sylvian fossa, are the predominant areas of this exudate. This predilection of exudate formation in the vicinity of the Sylvian fossa and of the second and third frontal gyrus, i.e. the areas which on the basis of findings in aphasia are regarded as the site of mental speech formation, is very noteworthy in regard to the clinical symptoms related to speech (mutism and verbigeration) which are very prominent in catatonia. Thus, on the basis of the frequency of symptoms related to speech and of the predilection sites for deposition of certain exudates, it is feasible to assume a relationship between clinical symptoms and disturbances in the pertinent part of the brain. However, it is not yet possible to prove this anatomically. Be this as it may, to my observation that the cloudiness of the arachnoidea in most cases does not extend to the above-mentioned parts of the frontal lobes I have to add that in all cases which I examined the pia could be removed easily from the surface of this part of the brain and that disturbances in continuity or other changes were never found in this area. I would like to remind the reader that in one case (VI) bone plates were embedded in the arachnoidea bilaterally over the frontal lobes, in areas of firm adherence between the dura and arachnoidea. In another case (II) the pia was adherent to the surface of the upper part of the frontal lobe, and in yet another (VII) the anterior point of the lower lobe was adherent to the dura—all facts which indicate that in areas adjoining the cerebral speech center, active processes of congestion and of exudate formation have taken place.

The microscopical examination of the brain cortex and of other parts of the brain in catatonia has not yielded me useful results, although I do not doubt that specific changes will also be demonstrated histologically in this disease when the normal and pathological histology of the brain has reached a more advanced stage. At present, definite results have not been obtained even in the well-known and repeatedly studied picture of progressive general paralysis.

Although the reported anatomical data may be fragmentary and their interpretation as yet insufficient to explain the disease process, I am of the opinion that they are not completely without value, since they afford an anatomical basis for this new form of disease and may stimulate its further study.

Finally we have to consider the behavior of extracerebral organs in catatonia. In the chapter on symptomatology I have already mentioned the frequent occurrence of edema in different parts of the body as a symptom in the sphere of trophic nerve functions. In the same chapter mention was made of clinical observations demonstrating a close relation and a high coincidence of the catatonic brain disease with other disturbances and complicating diseases, i.e. oligemia and chlorosis, and tuberculosis. Apart from other cases of catatonia in my practice which I did not report here and where tuberculosis was observed, 5 of the 7 above-described postmortems of patients with catatonia showed pulmonary tuberculosis, mostly in very advanced stages. Apart from this, tuberculosis is also frequently observed in other organs, especially in the mesenteric lymph nodes and in the intestinal wall, whereas tuberculosis of other organs without preexistent pulmonary tuberculosis has not been found in my studies.

Other tissue diseases occur similarly and—apart from oligemia—are not more frequent in catatonia than in other psychoses. It can be assumed that the reason for this extraordinarily close relationship between tuberculosis and catatonia lies in special characteristics of the catatonic disease process. These characteristics may be the general muscular stiffness and indolence, in a similar way as, on the one hand, precocious ossification of the rib cartilages and every process which limits the movements of the thorax have been found to cause pulmonary tuberculosis, while on the other hand systematic movements of the thorax, "inspiration gymnastics" are recommended to prevent the action of these detrimental tuberculosis promoting factors.

5

Diagnosis

The empirical material for the special description and delimitation of the disease having been collected and set out in the preceding chapters, we must now discuss the relationship between catatonia and other diseases and its most frequently occurring atypical forms. We can summarize the numerous data in the form of the following definition:

Catatonia is a brain disease with a cyclic, alternating course, in which the mental symptoms are, consecutively, melancholy, mania, stupor, confusion, and eventually dementia. One or more of these symptoms may be absent from the complete series of psychic "symptom-complexes". In addition to the mental symptoms, locomotor neural processes with the general character of convulsions occur as typical symptoms.

Thus defined, the disease follows, in respect of its clinical importance, closely upon the disease known as general paralysis of the insane with or without megalomania. In the latter disease there is also a cyclically changing alternation of symptoms, typically combined with symptoms of the motor nervous system, which in contrast to those in catatonia have the character of paralysis. Correlated with both these clinical types there is a third brain disease which shows typical mental symptoms and which also reveals a characteristically changing pattern of the mental symptom complex, but has no motor nervous symptoms. This last form, which usually involves admission to an institution in the stage of mania and which generally from this stage proceeds toward recovery, is usually indicated in the psychiatric nomenclature as mania or, in the complicated framework of other maniacal conditions, as simple or true mania. These disease forms with a cyclic course are in contrast to cases which, on the contrary, show an almost completely constant symptom complex or to cases with an irregular but not cyclically alternating symptom complex. Although the sphere of mental phenomena is most complicated and variegated, it can be determined with sufficient certainty that patients suffering from mental disease with a stable symptom complex (with the sole exception of insanity) behave in a characteristic manner in the limitation of their mental phenomena, i.e.

it appears that only a part of the psyche (mood, intelligence) is affected (partial mental disturbance), whereas in most cases with an alternating pattern all possible variations of mental disturbance are present, either simultaneously or consecutively (total or all-embracing mental disturbance). In addition it is interesting to note that in cases with a frequently changing, atypical character and without a cyclic course, a well-defined somatic disease can usually be found as a direct cause of the brain disease (sympathetic mental disturbance, e.g. mental disturbance after cardiac disease, or after typhoid or head injury).

According to these empirical and clinically important distinctions, catatonia is not a partial, but an extensive, more or less total mental disturbance. Since the disease does not develop after a certain somatic disease, but at most on the basis of a disease tendency (anemia), and since it does not have an irregular but a *cyclic* and *typical* alternation of the symptoms, it can be used as a basis for a general distinction between idiopathic and somatogenic mental diseases.

Catonia shows marked variations in the manner in which the disease develops in individual patients. It may be possible to distinguish a total and a simple form of the disease according to the larger or smaller number of typical symptoms of the complete mental syndrome present during the consecutive stages. An epileptoid, tetanic, choreatic, cataleptic or indifferent form may be distinguished when locomotor neural symptoms are especially prominent or only weakly developed. However, since there is no correlation between the above two series of distinctions, these are not suitable for a correct subdivision of the disease. All that can be done at present is to distinguish severe or complicated and mild or simple cases, depending on whether the mental and motor phenomena, which are to be regarded as signs of irritation, are very prominent or less developed. A form known from the institutions (which is therefore very frequent and may thus be regarded as typical) is that type which until now was known as atonic melancholy or *mélancholie avec stupeur*. After initial symptoms of simple melancholy, the patient develops the condition of stupor—during which a few locomotor symptoms can always be recognized—and this eventually leads either to recovery or to insanity. As mentioned above, epileptic convulsions, which occur during the earliest development of the disease, when people around the patient do not yet notice any mental disease, are usually not even reported to the physicians at the institution. In the same way transient conditions of excitation and sudden, short-lived joy are rather frequent but at the same time so transitory that they do not alter the course of the disease. These typical cases, which in the classification so far used have already been regarded as a separate group, can be designated as the simple form *(catatonia mitis)*.

Subsequently the second group is made up of cases where prolonged, more or less marked mania develops after symptoms of melancholy. These cases are often cured before the stage of permanent stupor, and in the conventional diagnostic nomenclature they were usually designated as simple mania. These severe, and mentally more developed, cases also include those where the locomotor symptoms do not consist of a single or a few attacks, but are more prolonged and have attracted the attention of the physician, so that these cases are treated as curiosa or as irregular complications. This is the form called *catatonia gravis*.

Finally, a third group can perhaps be constituted from special cases where the signs of irritation are not confined to the first half of the disease course, but tend to appear also subsequently, then usually combined with remissions or intermissions. This is the protracted form of catatonia.

The differential diagnosis is usually not difficult when the observation material is more or less complete. The characteristic symptoms of this disease form are so prominent at all stages that there cannot be more than faint doubts, at least if the observation has been thorough. An isolated attack of convulsions which is regarded as epilepsy, eclampsia, apoplexia, meningitis or encephalitis and which can occur either during complete health or after "a long period of a somewhat peculiar mental behavior," leaving no signs of paresis, excitation with agitation, or severe depression, is always followed by periods of unmotivated taciturnity, at least by a tendency to fixed positions, and will in such cases also be combined with negativistic peculiarities. If recovery does not occur in this stage, the complete development of the stage of stuporous atonicity will follow. We may also note, in a patient designated as melancholic, the presence of a markedly pathetic behavior and a strangely fixed position of the body; in these cases we can predict with almost apodictic certainty the beginning of atonicity. When a patient who has previously spoken develops permanent taciturnity, combined with fixed positions of the body and the extremities, there can be almost no doubt that this is a case of catatonia, whatever the previous history. Only two other possibilities have to be taken into account in these cases, when an anamnesis is not available, i.e. apathy with fixed habits in infantile insanity, and the same syndrome, but transiently, in mental disturbances after somatic diseases. But here usually an exact observation will lead to the diagnosis without knowledge of the anamnesis. In the first case the cretinoid development of the head and body will afford the distinction, and in the second case the apathy, which is only apparent and which immediately changes into a reaction after passive attempts at movements. Real difficulties exist in only two aspects, in the first place during the first half of the disease course, when the occurrence of neuromotor symptoms has not been observed and when there is as yet no persistent taciturnity. In this respect we must realize that complete atonicity is only a very high degree of development of this symptom, and that unmotivated silence or even only the sparing use of words, with daily intervals, may precede or even replace atonicity. In many cases the characteristic symptom of pathetic behavior and the unmotivated repetition of words or sentences may be of help.

The second case of a difficulty in diagnosis exists when a patient who has been melancholic and sparing with words during a long period of time manifests no neuromotor symptoms, and when this is followed by the development of marked taciturnity without a prominent tendency to fixed positions and without important changes or increases in the preexisting intellectual content of the melancholy. It may be wondered whether the melancholy which has been observed up to this moment has been a simple initial melancholy which changes into atonicity without an intervening phase with signs of irritation, or whether this has been a partial and permanent disturbance of the mood where the almost complete taciturnity has to be regarded not as a new symptom but as an increase in the previously observed sparing use of words. For the time being it is not possible to resolve this problem; the solution will come when other, possibtly neuropathic means of distinction point the way in one of these directions. It is possible, even probable, that this is a case where in pathology, as in other natural areas, a transition occurs of one form to another, preventing an exact delimitation.

In the large majority of cases the main symptoms are so fully developed that it is impossible to mistake catatonia for another form of disease, once we have recognized and acquainted ourselves with this form.

Even when we disregard the specially developed condition of atonic melancholy, repetition of words and speeches, stereotyped gestures and habits and negativistic expressions of the will are such striking symptoms and are so characteristic of the disease form that even in the presence of the most far-reaching reluctance against construction of symptomatologic syndromes the special analogy and the special place of such cases cannot be denied. On the other hand the diagnosis of this disease form in one of its earliest stages and the prognosis and anamnesis are so easy to survey and so important clinically that we would be sacrificing practical usefulness to hypercriticality if we were not to separate these cases clinically and in practice.

6

Prognosis

With regard to prognosis, catatonia shows a contrast to general paralysis of the insane, with or without megalomania. Whereas the prognosis in GPI is known, and justly so, to be extremely bad, the prognosis of all forms of catatonia is by no means hopeless. This is true concerning both the possibility of a cure and life expectancy. In the above-reported experiences, grouped together in the scheme of atonic melancholy, the prognosis is fair, this being true not only for cases with absence or only slight development of signs of irritation, but also for cases with very marked convulsions and agitation, recovery occurring even when unpleasant secondary signs of irritation or of feebleness are present. Recovery is relatively so frequent that this gratifying contrast with paralysis, where it is even doubtful whether a cure is at all possible, must be recognized immediately. In this context the following case will be quoted, where recovery occurred after only 3 months.

26. Case history

Siegmund X., secretary in a regional court of justice in G., 43 years old. Weak constitution, previously generally healthy, but during recent years had suffered from varices and ulcers of the legs. He worked very hard, was happily married, and had six children one of which died during Easter 1867. He had guilt feelings of having neglected this child and was irritable and very gloomy during a long period. The following summer he had to replace a colleague, and during this time he had an extremely onerous work load.

In November of the same year he again suffered from furuncles and subsequent lymphangitis of the lower legs, accompanied with slight bronchial catarrh and followed by very high fever. He again became highly irritable, and during this change in mood he turned, at the beginning of December, into a complete insomniac. On the second day of this period of insomnia his wife noted his pathetically exalted speech, with a preferential use of diminutives. The following night a physician who was called in found the whole family hastily dressed, crying at the side of his bed. The patient himself appeared to be quiet (extasis). He declared in a joyful tone of voice that he had thought about his disease and that he was convinced that he would die of blood poisoning. He was calmed by the physician, and the following day he said that he had been excited, had experienced the sensation that his head had turned into a barrel, had smelled corpses, etc. During the same day attacks of excitation recurred, and at night he showed very marked changes in his manner of speaking, and declared that he was "wonderfully healthy." After he had slept for two hours, a state of extreme extasis appeared: "Such a nice sleep I have never had in my whole life." He had the feeling of having been in other regions, in a world of ghosts. He wished his wife could also be so happy (quoted by his wife when she described the development of the disease). The excitation increased on the following day—he declared that a miracle had befallen him, he had died, and God had sanctified his body and resurrected him. He did not need or wish to sleep any more. Those two hours of slumber had been exactly enough. A peculiar repetition of these words became striking. When his wife contradicted his statements, he developed an aversion to her. His behavior became very strange. At times he lay completely motionless, without reaction, and with fixed gaze. Sometimes he laughed so loudly, without apparent motivation, that his whole body shook; this was combined with grimacing (epileptic or choreiformic convulsions). He would often say without any particular reason: "That is too ridiculous." He did not want to see his doctor, and when the latter wanted to give him an enema he resisted: "his body was a sanctified body, he did not want to have his body touched—that would be profanity . . . " Initially he accepted the suggestion that he go outside to recuperate, and he even put his clothes on and strutted proudly about the house, despite his sick leg.

On the 6th day of the mental alteration (counting from the insomnia) he was admitted to the institute and was placed with the restless patients.

He was of weak physical build, of average height, with a scrophulous constitution and tuberculous appearance. At first he behaved quietly and showed slight euphoria. When the pain caused by the furuncles disappeared after the application of moist bandages, he even became somewhat cheerful. When he was moved to a quiet ward on account of his continued calm behavior, he became negativistic and irritable, spoke about nitrogen being spread in this new room, and at night he developed a tendency to fixed positions. While he was lying in bed because of the ulcer on his lower leg, he remained stretched out, without speaking or reacting, all the time keeping his head slightly above the pillow (tetaniform cramp), his hands folded, and his eyes focused on one point (atonicity). The whole night he lay quietly in this manner. The following day he now and then spoke excitedly. From that time he showed very changeable behavior with rapid transitions, at times quiet (but then without lucidity) and at times very confused in his speech and wishes, singing or shouting loudly. During these periods he suffered hallucinations with all the senses, especially smell and sight; he talked extensively about situations which rose up before his eyes in his hallucinations, etc. At times he spoke in a mysterious fashion with unusual forms of speech, and he manifested paranoic ideas, in which "the Lodge" played a prominent part. Sometimes he screamed and appeared to be in a cramplike fixed position, and he would then often repeat a certain word, e.g. "house rules, house rules," or complete sentences. These were often constructed in such a way that they started with the phrase "house rule," and this was then followed by a series of more or less inarticulate sounds, and finally by the words "little father" (verbigeration). He often rolled about in his bed, but without using his hands, as if he had cramps, until he was soaked in sweat. Finally, as the third phase of this alternating state, he developed a condition characterized by a tendency to fixed positions, during which he lay stiffly extended, without reactions or speech, while he pulled at the bedclothes. During a certain period it was possible to observe a fourth phase, as it were, which was designated very aptly by the head nurse as a "quiet attack." The patient then lay in his fixed position and gnashed his teeth (mandibular cramps). These attacks occurred irregularly during the day and night.

Initially the patient received opium 0.05. This gave him a better night. He was then given opium with the same amount of ZnO, one dose in the morning and one at night, and later a double dose of opium.

In the first part of the fourth week the attacks began to desist, and after two months them it was possible to hold a sensible conversation with the patient; he then expressed normal feelings, but still did not appear to have a clear understanding of the attacks which still occurred, despite the fact that his consciousness was never decreased as in epilepsy. Once, for example, to the question why he did not suppress an attack which was accompanied with convulsive movements of the whole body, he replied that "in the past I had been a hunchback."

In the first part of the fourth week the attacks began to desist, and after two months the patient was able to be moved to the recovery ward. His memory of the abnormal condition which he had passed through remained vague. When he became quieter his nutritional state improved. A month later, this patient, who had been in a very bad condition when admitted, was dismissed from the institute, strong and in radiant health. His mental well-being was permanent, and the prognosis of the case remained good despite the absence of a clear recollection of his attacks and convulsions. This was demonstrated by the fact that 5 years later this patient himself arranged for a mental patient from a family with whom he was friendly to be admitted to the institute.

Regarding the single factors which determine the prognosis of a possible cure in a certain case, my experience with catatonia agrees with the general theses which have been established for mental illnesses. However, in my opinion, the great importance ascribed in other diseases to the occurrence of cramplike symptoms and convulsions in individual patients does not hold true in cases which can be diagnosed as catatonia. Among prognostic factors derived from the anamnesis, masturbation is usually regarded as very unfavorable. However, masturbation should not only be regarded as an etiological factor, for it also has symptomatologic importance, i.e. it is the expression of a pathological irritation of the genital organs which persists after the appearance of the catatonia and is one of the causes of the latter's persistence. Thus, masturbation has no especially unfavorable prognostic importance, since the cause of this promoting and accompanying symptom can be eliminated surgically (by catheterization) or by means of drugs or a diet. In addition, forbidding the patient to masturbate on moral grounds plus surveillance can be used successfully in the suppression of this harmful factor. In other diseases a long duration is an unfavorable prognostic factor, and this is also true for catatonia. However, in this disease more than in any other clinical form of disease there is still a good possibility of recovery even after a long period, provided that no other adverse factors are present or appear, such as concentration of the intellectual symptoms on a particular delusion, complication with unfavorable somatic diseases, as, for example, pulmonary tuberculosis, advanced age, etc. Concentration of the delirium on a limited group of ideas or even on one "idée fixe" is a definitely unfavorable symptom, but in this regard the idée fixe should not be mistaken for undifferentiated emotions. An unchanging melancholy in mood and feelings does not in itself worsen the prognosis of catatonia. Similarly, according to my observations, a factor which is otherwise regarded as especially adverse, i.e. dirtiness, even the patient's playing with his own stools, and coprophagy, does not have the same serious prognostic significance as in other disease forms.

Considering the prognosis of survival, we must first remark that catatonia is probably a directly lethal psychosis, just as this is stated of paralysis in contrast to most other mental diseases. Whereas in other forms of psychosis complicating somatic diseases, exhaustion after refusal of food, or excessive excitation are the causes of death while the brain process itself is usually not apt to lead to this result, in catatonia death may occur as the last stage, as it were, the highest developmental phase of atonicity, i.e. the outcome of the disease itself. The condition of atonicity may be regarded as a kind of vita minima if it does not appear in the initial stages as a more or less intensive and evident tension. It may be compared with syncope and lethargy, and when it has persisted for a long time it seems on the one hand to be able, without local disturbances and as its own anatomical basis, to cause a complete breakdown of the vital functions, while on the other, it may cause damaging factors, which in themselves are not of major importance, to lead to death.

The frequent complication with pulmonary tuberculosis is one of the unfavorable factors of the prognosis of survival, since its seriousness is an additional threat cast on the period beyond recovery from the mental disease.

This is the most suitable point at which to discuss the outcome in cases where a period of noisy or otherwise significant activity (more or less maniacal) is followed by a longer period of complete external quiet, but without a return of lucid awareness, even without memory of the period of mental disturbances. In other forms of disease the latter is rightly demanded as a prerequisite sign of a complete and certain convalescence. It is noteworthy that, as reported earlier, I have observed especially in catatonia, a strikingly persistent negation or absence of a subjective recollection of the disease. I was often unable to decide whether to declare a patient fit, even though active disturbances had been absent for a long time and even though there was a tendency and capacity for regular and prolonged employment, or a normal emotional relationship with the relatives had been reestablished. However, I have been happy to note repeatedly in these cases—when the patient had to be discharged from the institute due to external circumstances—that the improvement increased despite the absence of subjective insight into the disease, or that the cure persisted and no relapse occurred. The last-reported case history also belongs in this category. In this case I myself, on the basis of previous experience, had arranged for the patient to be discharged since, due to his individual peculiarities, I believed that a prolonged stay in the institute might easily have led to renewed emotional irritation. From this case it was possible to derive the principle that catatonics can, under certain circumstances, be released earlier, or at least with greater confidence, than patients with other mental diseases under the same conditions. Such patients can be directed from specialist treatment to convalescence at home. This is possible when all active signs of irritation have disappeared and when the patient expresses his desire to resume his normal occupation and is lucid enough to do this, or when his normal emotional relationship with his relatives has been restored.

As regards the general risk of a relapse, this is on the whole relatively small in catatonia. Among the patients whom I have observed, none has fallen ill again to date. However, in some cases slight mental disturbances had for a long time preceded the disease, without resulting in the patient's being admitted to the institute. It is not possible to decide whether during these periods they were already suffering from catatonia.

In this chapter on the prognosis of mental disturbances we must also ask ourselves what can be expected from the offspring of persons who have suffered from catatonia, i.e. whether their children are born with a special predisposition for mental diseases, and if so, for which type. This is perhaps related to the question of whether catatonics are of normal fertility. In my experience, people who have suffered from catatonia are in general normally fertile, since in a number of cases I have noticed that they have had children. With regard to the propensity of children of ex-catatonics for mental diseases, my empirical observations are for the time being naturally insufficient. After the form of the disease has been established a new generation must be observed before definitive data can be obtained. Nevertheless, on the basis of observations conducted in East Prussia, and taking into account the relatively very isolated character of the province's population, I can state that this propensity is probably not marked. This is based on the fact that if a striking disposition did exist, I would have observed this among the patients admitted to the institute in Allenberg and among my other contacts. We must thus safeguard catatonia from its inclusion in the French concept of *degeneration*, which unfortunately is already starting to creep into the German literature. This also holds for the disease entity for which I earlier proposed the name of *hebephrenia* (juvenile insanity)*; I wish to mention this here as a clarification of the work of my colleague Hecker.

---

*VIRCHOW. *Arch. f. Path. Anat.*, etc., 1870.

7

Therapy

The further we enter into the distinction of nosological-clinical entities, the greater the need becomes to collect rich observation material in order to build a solid basis for our considerations. This is especially true when each successive entity is closely related in special points to its predecessors. However, when a new form of disease is proposed, the possibility of accumulating empirical data and the subsequent scrutiny of these to determine scientific facts in accord with other nosological viewpoints are negatively correlated; moreover, this is a very slow process. I naturally paid prime attention to the diagnostic delimitation when collecting my clinical experiences, since the reliability and the interest of all additional investigations into the disease depend on the solidity of this pillar of medical science. I therefore set myself first to collect and arrange the symptomatological and anatomicopathological material; only later was I to concentrate on the more practical subjects of prognosis and therapy, and the latter only at a late stage, since the proposal of a new disease form calls for abandoning old forms of treatment and performing multidimensional and precise experimental research to devise the correct therapy. These arguments were the reason that in this first treatise on my clinical experiences the chapters on the nosological matters have been more extensively worked out, while the later chapters on the more practical nosological relationships are less detailed. Another reason for the brevity of these chapters is that the later case reports, which were chosen to demonstrate practical points of interest, are of patients some of whom are still under observation; it is obviously impossible to give detailed information on these recent cases. In the final chapter on therapy I wish to confine myself to brief indications; more detailed discussions will be published in a later monograph, where I shall be able to present a statistical survey of a full set of clinical forms after presenting a few other, partly new, clinical forms of disease.

The main therapeutic question in psychiatry is whether patients with catatonia can with advantage be treated at home or whether immediate institutionalization is better. My experience leaves no doubt that for the best results, early admission to a good institution is essential. In cases with maniacal attacks a rapid transfer is required in the interest of the safety of both the patient and the people around him, for all sorts of intolerable situations are liable to crop up, including attempts of suicide or murder. In addition, the basic idea of a rational therapy during the developmental stage is, as in most other psychoses, to prevent all emotional excitement and all stimulation of the senses and of the imagination. Even in cases with a relatively quiet course, where at least in the initial stage the outward calm is mostly only apparent and probably the result of an overpowering of the psyche by external impressions, attempts to keep the patients in the usual conditions at home have, in my experience, not ended well. In most cases the refusal of food necessitates the intervention of a physician with good technical training, and this in itself is reason enough for hospitalization. But apart from this, the mental upheaval caused by moving the patient with mild catatonia from his home to the institution can sometimes be such a strong positive factor that after a relatively short time marked improvement can be obtained, even if a complete cure is not achieved. To confirm this I refer the reader to case 26 and to the remark in the preceding chapter regarding the discharge of patients.

In respect to the details of treatment, I must emphasize that there is no specific drug or method and that, as in other mental diseases, the preliminary experiences are on the whole rather negative. After repeated, and temporarily promising, attempts with various drugs and methods we always have to return to an anticipatory procedure, consisting in eliminating external stimuli during the first half of the disease and in cautiously modifying mental impressions and stimuli in the second half; this method certainly has an active and positive content. Among the drugs which have become accepted by long usage, the series of tonics has been most reliable and was most frequently successful. These drugs appear to be indicated in catatonia due to the type of the disease process and the general somatic condition. In some cases which were cured the use of iron and quinine combined with a diet and with a regulation of the daily routine of the patient (when necessary implemented against his will) appear to have contributed greatly to the favorable outcome. An anemic condition of the skin and the visible mucosae in general is very frequent in catatonia and sometimes excessive; in addition amenorrhea and chlorosis, or factors causing debility, form the indication for this treatment. However, in many cases where the above factors were less prominent, a similar treatment increasing the tonus turned out to be effective.

According to such experiences, it is self-evident that the drugs and methods which are based on opposite view points—debilitating treatment—which were formerly widely accepted and extensively applied in all psychoses, are absolutely contraindicated in catatonia. My experiences are in accordance with the warnings issued by all modern psychiatrists against the use of debilitating treatment in all forms of mental disease, including all varieties of catatonia. However, despite this warning, repeated almost ad nauseam, against the use of bloodletting in general, against laxatives, and the withdrawal of fluids by means of a diet or taking the waters at spas, we observe again and again in the institutions cases where in the anamnesis an important part is played by venesection, or by long and tiring journeys to cold-water spas, since the patient or his family makes the mistake of wishing to avoid the asylum. For the sake of completeness I wish to stress that venesection is contraindicated even in cases with a very rapid development of true catatonia. In numerous cases where before admission to an institution the outmoded practice of bloodletting was performed, not an improvement was obtained but on the contrary a deterioration. In the same way, visits to a spa and taking the waters without the prerequisite of well-considered action (i.e. elimination or moderation of mental and emotional stimuli) are so frequent among subsequently institutionalized catatonics that their general damaging effect may be considered certain, even though there are rare cases where one of these treatments may have apparently helped, in which case the event dies hard and is held up as a special instance.

In the same way I can confirm the total ineffectiveness, at any stage, of those superior medicaments of the old school—stibium tartrate in small doses and blistering drugs applied to the skull and head (stibium tartrate ointment, croton oil). According to former usage in the East Prussian and other institutions, a certain treatment was adopted as a last resort when all else had failed, the disease threatened to become chronic, and the patients were about to be dismissed as incurable; this consisted in shaving the head and applying "pustule ointment." However, the increasingly common sight of hairless pates in the institutions did not indicate brilliant results from this method. On the other hand, spontaneous cures were regularly noted in the course of the years among "incurables" who had not received a tonsure.

From these opposing methods of roboration and debilitation we come to the third main group of drugs and methods, i.e. those which cause alterations in behavior. Among these, narcotics and drugs acting on the nerves must be taken into consideration. Belladonna and ZnO are used because of the spastic character of the disease, but usually without a particularly reliable effect. Potassium bromide appeared to be indicated because of the high incidence of irritation of the genital organs; its use was not without effect on this symptom, but as far as we can perceive it showed no definite influence on the convulsivity or the general pathological condition. It seems advisable to perform further trials with this and with the two preceding drugs. Special indications will probably be found which will lead to good results in special cases and in cases with a specific course.

Opium has been tried several times, without any effect, in cases where a prominent melancholic mood caused a resemblance or relation to dysthymia (so-called true or simple melancholy), which formed an indication for this antidepressive drug.

On the other hand, it seems we have methods of very great therapeutic importance in faradic and galvanic electricity, although for the time being the indications have not yet been worked out, and in many cases the action might be explained more on the basis of mental than of physiopathological effects. In some cases the use of galvanic electricity has also had a markedly adverse effect, with excitation and deterioration of the mood. This method appears to me to be of special importance in catatonia in regard to the predisposition for pulmonary tuberculosis. The inhibiting effect of the slow muscle action on the dilatation of the lung alveoli and on the blood circulation in the thorax (and consequently on the intracranial circulation) may be interrupted by faradization of the thoracic muscles.

Subject Index

"Abulie" 27
Abusive language 18, 26
Affective reactions, violent 10
Aggressivity 48
Amenorrhea 94
Anemia 55, 84
Anorexia 51
Anticipating procedures 94
Apathetic 10, 22, 40
Apathy 18, 21, 22, 25, 26, 36, 42, 43, 85
Apoplexia 85
Appetite 15
Arachnoidea 74, 75, 76, 77, 78, 79, 80
Atonia 24, 25, 26
Atonic melancholia 8, 23, 25, 26, 49, 51, 54, 84, 87
Antonicity 20, 22, 31–34, 36, 38, 40, 42, 45, 46, 48, 50, 51, 58, 67, 71, 85, 86, 88, 90
Autopsies, summary
  See: Postmortems

Behavioral aberrations 10
Belladonna 95
Bowel movements 14, 15
  coprophagy 90
  obstipation 62
  severe constipation 11

Camisards 57
Cataleptic state 8
Cataleptiform incidents 20
Catatonia 6, 9, 17, 21, 27, 29, 30–34, 39, 40, 42, 46, 48, 49, 51–53, 54–57, 59, 78, 79, 80, 81, 84, 88–91

definition 83
endemic occurrence 56, 58
epidemic occurrence 56
Cerebrovascular syphilis
  See: General paralysis of the insane,
       Tabes Dorsalis
Chlorosis 51, 55, 80, 94
Chloreiform
  facial tics 10
  muscle activity 11
  seizures 14, 26
Cholera infection 17
Coarse language 22
Cold-water cure 17
Compulsion 18, 20
Confabulation 41
Confusion 21, 29, 32, 41, 43, 45, 83
Contractures of the musculature 23
Convulsions 19, 21, 26, 36, 38, 41, 50, 57, 77, 83, 87, 89
Convulsive states 20
Cramp
  in central nervous speech path, 41
  "snout" 43, 50
  tetaniform 88
Cyclic pattern 33

Debilitating treatment contraindicated 94, 95
Decreased sensibility 51
Deliriun 37, 49
Delusions 33–37, 43, 47, 55, 69
  of grandeur 8, 9, 11, 27, 37
  religious 55, 58, 60

Dementia 16, 20, 21, 22, 32, 33, 41, 43, 46, 77
  stupida 8
  terminal 8, 9, 31, 32, 45, 79
  total 14
Depression 8, 10, 13, 16, 23, 32, 43, 45, 85
  depressive agitation 20
  despondency 23
Deterioration in intelligence 13
Deterioration, mental 14, 26
Dirtiness 36, 90
Discharge of patients 94
Disturbance(s)
  of intelligence 34
  of thought processes 38
  of will or action 34
Drugs, use of 94
  cupr. sulph. ammon. 22
  opium 89, 95
  opium with ZnO 89
  potassium bromide 95
  ZnO 95
Dysthymia 55

Eclampsia 85
Edema 16, 51, 80
Electricity, use of
  galvanic current 42
  galvanic and faradic 95, 96
  galvanization 44
Encephalitis 85
Epidermal crusts 52
Epilepsy
  epileptic attack 77
  epileptic cramps 69
  epileptiform attack 50
  epileptoid form 84
Excessive sweating 15
Excessive talkativeness 20
Excitation with agitation 85
Extasis 88

Fantasies 18
  depressive 13
  religious 20
Fear 13
Fetor ex ore 52
Flexibilatas cerea
  See: Waxen flexibility
"Flight of ideas" 41, 46

Gardening activities 13
General paralysis of the insane (GPI) 2, 6, 7, 27, 37, 48, 53, 54, 74, 77, 78, 87
  paralytic insanity 52
  Tabes Dorsalis 8
GPI
  See: General paralysis of the insane

Hallucinations 11, 20–22, 25, 34, 35, 38, 42, 43, 47, 88, 89
Headache 43
Hebephrenia
  See: Juvenile insanity
Hematomas of ear 52
Heredity 53, 67
Hostility 18
Hypochondriac(al) 23, 32, 33, 35
  hysterical-hypochondriacal 19
Hysteria 50

"Idée fixe" 90
Illusions 39
Impairment, general mental activity 13
Impulse to undress 19
Incessant talking 16
Indifferent form 84
Insanity 29, 30, 33, 34, 39, 69, 83
  complicated by catalepsy 20
  complicated by muscle spasms 27
  infantile 85
  temporary 21
  tension-insanity 29
Insecurity, feeling of 13
Insomnia 87, 88
Institutionalization 93
Intellectual exertion 54, 55

Jansenism 57
Juvenile insanity 6, 92

Language, abusive 26
Lawyers 54
Locomotor
  apparatus 27
  functions 22
  neural processes 83
  neural symptoms 84
  symptoms 84

Mania 18, 20, 23, 26, 31–33, 36, 38, 42, 46, 48, 50, 67, 68, 83, 84
Maniacal 34, 37, 38, 39, 40, 46, 60, 71, 91, 94
Manic
  outbursts 21, 22
  phase 19, 30, 48
  state 8, 25, 26
Masturbation 35, 37, 38, 54, 90
Megalomania 34, 37, 47, 74–76, 78, 87
Melancholia 16, 23, 25, 27, 30, 31, 33, 35, 38, 42, 43, 45, 47, 57, 68, 74, 84, 86, 95
  combined with mental deficiency 29
  "melancolie avec stupeur" 27, 84
  See also: Depression
Melancholic disorders 3
  agitation 42, 43
  atonicity 9
  attonita 8, 27
  stupida 27
Meningitis 85
Merchants 54
Mood 13, 14, 18, 29, 30, 37, 41–43, 47, 55, 60, 84, 86, 87
Movements
  passive 12
  spastic 27
Murder 94
Musculature, weak 15
Mute 22
  mutism 80
  speechlessness 27
  taciturnity 41, 42, 64, 75, 85, 86

Negative voluntary movement 26
Negativism 47, 49
Negativistic 85
Negativity 46
Nervous excitation 17, 18
Noncommunicative 10
Nutritional state, poor 24

Obsessive need to undress 21
Oligemia 51, 55, 80
Onanism 11, 22

Paralysis 87
  general progressive 76, 79
  progressive 77
"Paralytic mental illness" 27

Paresis 27, 85
Pathetic behavior 85
Pathological pathos 39
Perspire, tendency to 15
Phosphorylated ether, treatment with 12
Physical activities 13
Physical force 18
Postmortems 59, 61, 65, 67, 69, 70–76
  review of anatomical findings 78–81
  specific histologic changes 80
Psychic deterioration 14
Psychopathological process 3
Psychopathological state 3
Pulmonary tuberculosis 52, 81, 90

Rage, uncontrollable 22, 75
Refusing food, phenomenon 48
Repetition of words, unmotivated 85
Repressed 13

Seizures
  clonic 26
  convulsive 14, 16
  convulsive fits 22
  convulsive type fits 22
  convulsivelike disorders 17
  semitonic spastic conditions 22
  See also: Convulsions
Sensory perception 14, 18, 22
Sensory response 12, 15
Sexual overstimulation 54
"Snout cramp" 43, 50
Somatic symptoms 50
  disturbances 51
Somnambulism 22
Somnolence 37
Spasmodic conditions
  flexibilitas cerea 50
  cramps 50, 51
  tetanic cramps 50
  trismus 50
Spasms
  muscle (arms and mouth) 11
  muscular twitchings 14
  "snout-spasm" 22
Spastic
  contractions, of facial and cervical musculature 10
  muscle activity 19
  signs 27

Stereotyped movements 49, 50
Stereotypically performed movements 20, 70
"Stupidite" 27
Stupor 8, 24, 29, 83, 84
Suicide, 31, 32, 51, 53, 94
Syphilitic infection 14
   secondary stage 14, 29

Tabes Dorsalis 8
Teachers 54, 55
Tetanic contractions 21
   form 84
Tetany 6
   and psychosis 6
Theologians 54
Tonic contractions
   of back muscles 14
Tonic-mental disorder (Spannungs-Irresein) 27

Tuberculosis 81, 90

Urinary incontinence 22, 63, 64
   nocturnal 22

Vascular tonus in extremities 14
   with edema 14
Verbigeration 41, 46, 58, 70, 80, 89
   talkativeness 18
   verbal diarrhea 21
   verbocity 41
Vesania katatonica (catatonia) 27
Violence, acts of 34
"Voluntary Function and Muscle Activity" 28

Waxen flexibility 8, 9, 17, 26, 36, 51
   immobile 49
   rigidity of body 22

Author Index

Ackernecht, E. xiv
Albers, Johann A. 31, 32
Arndt, Rudolf G. 6

Baillarger, J. x, xi, xiii, 8, 29
Baruk, H. xv
Bayle, H. L. x, xii
Beneke, E. x
Bernhardi, Dr. vii
Bismarck, Otto von viii
Burrows, G. xi, 29
Burton, Robert ix

Calmeil, L. F. x, xii, 56
Chaslin xiv
Chiarugi, Vincenzo ix
Conolly, J. x
Cullen, William ix

De Boor, W. xiv
de Jong, Herman H. xv
de Sauvage, Boissier Francois ix
de Tours, Moreau J. x
Descartes, Renée ix

Ellenberger, Henri ix
Esquirol, Jean Etienne x

Falrét, J. x, xiii, xiv, 3
Ferrus, G. x
Feuchtersleben, E. x

Georget, E.J. x
Goethe, Johann Wofgang von viii

Griesinger, W. x, xi, xiii, 8, 29
Guislain xi, 8

Halle, J.N. 56
Haslam, J. xi
Hecker, Ewald viii, xi, xiv, xv
Heinroth, Johann C.A. x
Hill, Robert G. x
Hippocrates ix

Ideler, Carl W. x

Jacobi, Maximilian x
Jelliffe, Smith Ely xv
Jessen, W. 56

Kant, Immanuel viii
Karaagac, Ishan A. xvi
Katzenstein, Rafael xiv
Kelp 29, 41
König, E. 31
Kraepelin, Emil xiv, xv, 8

Leubuscher 56
Linné, Carl von viii, ix

Meding 31
Meyer, Adolf xv, 77
Meynert, Theodor xiv
Morel, Benedict Auguste xi, xii

Nasse, Friedrich x
Neisser, Clemens xv
Neumann, Heinrich xi, xii, xiii

Pinel, Philippe ix, x
Platter, Felix ix
Prichard, James C. x

Reil, Johann C. x
Rush, Benjamin ix, x

Schule, Heinrich xiv
Seglas, Jules xiv
Seguin, Edward x
Spengler 57
Spielmann, J.R. 31, 32

Sydenham, Thomas ix

Tuke, William ix

Virchow, Rudolf, L.K. vii, 6, 73
Voisin, Felix x

Willis, Thomas ix

Zacchia, Paolo ix
Zeller, Ernest xi, 8
Zilboorg, Gregory xiv, xv